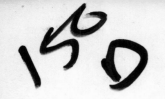

LOOK YOUNGER LOOK PRETTIER

beauty through diet and yoga techniques

LOOK YOUNGER LOOK PRETTIER

beauty through diet and yoga techniques

by Virginia Castleton Thomas

Designed and Produced by Charles F. Beck

RODALE PRESS, INC.   BOOK DIVISION   EMMAUS, PA. 18049

Standard Book Number 0-87857-018-7
Library of Congress Card No. 70-190201
COPYRIGHT 1972
by Virginia Castleton Thomas

PRINTED IN U.S.A.

B-546

FIFTH PRINTING — APRIL, 1975

LOOK YOUNGER - LOOK PRETTIER

TABLE OF CONTENTS

To Joy Gorin
who introduced me to
Yoga-American style.

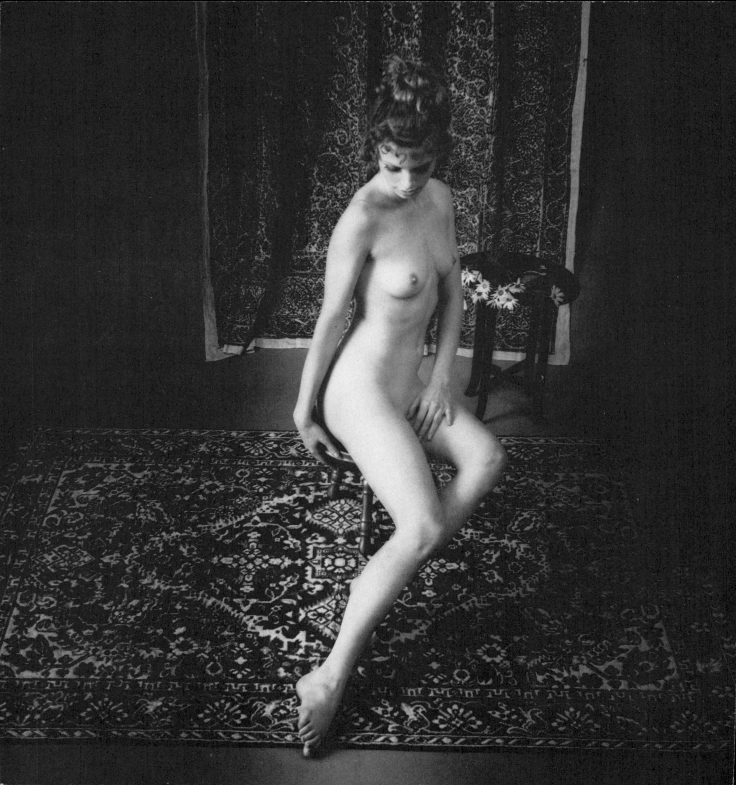

CHAPTER ONE - NEW BODIES FOR OLD

IF new bodies to replace worn, ill and neglected ones were for sale, how many of us would grab our checkbooks and shout, "I'll take one; how much?"

Practically everyone would succumb to this offer.

While it may not be possible to buy such a body, it is possible to gain a new body. It can be had without reaching for a checkbook, but rather by using the body we already have. Yet, when one discovers that he must do the remaking himself, how many are going to lose interest? How many will be willing to give a few minutes a day toward restoring the body to fine working condition, health, and beauty?

The regular practice of Hatha Yoga can present you with a body that has been changed for the better, just as if you had followed a design for rebuilding or remaking a home or any other structure. Yoga exercises minimize the work in creating a perfect figure, a composed mind, and an overall sense of glowing good health.

What do we mean by good health? Good health indicates an absence of disease and the many disabilities of a prematurely aging body. The faithful practice of Yoga helps to nip in the bud ailments brought about by neglect and disuse of the body.

The movements of this practice can also re-establish the vitality that has been lost through sedentary living. Correctly performed, Yoga exercises are not tiring. Unlike more demanding calisthenic movements, fifteen minutes with Yoga leaves one refreshed and relaxed.

Yoga teaches that one cannot be a week-end exercise enthusiast and still avoid the pitfalls that await the sedentary person. Two hectic days of golf, tennis, swimming, or volley ball will not bring about the steady state of good health that a shorter *daily* exercise period will.

Exercise is like vitamin C in some respects. Neither can be stored up for later use; they must be taken daily. A quarter hour of Yoga exercises every day is far more beneficial than two straight days of concentrated sport. In fact, the concentrated, all-or-nothing method of exercise is alien to Yogic principle. Easy, gentle, but steady use of the body will bring far greater rewards, provided a person cares enough about the body to devote a small fraction of the day's time to restoration.

Beauty of body, grace of movement, and inner health will all come from these simple exercises that have been adapted to our Western society from their original Eastern culture.

The body is a beautiful mechanism. Its ability to perform an almost infinite variety of tasks far exceeds that of any bit of machinery. Therefore, it is the duty of everyone to develop his body to the highest degree of perfection and to maintain it by daily care. This is a very practical dedication, for by being knowledgeable and concerned about the body, many uncomfortable days of illness can be avoided.

Statistics show the advantages of using the body to side-step the ills of sedentary life. Members of the Garment Workers Union in New York City enjoy outstandingly good health, because of the physical nature of their work. Because they flex their bodies in continual exertion, they have a lower sickness rate than other workers who merely check the garments or attend to clerical duties.

Hatha Yoga is a very practical science, a complete re-education of the mind and body. Though dealing mainly with improvements to the body through gentle physical movements, Hatha Yoga teaches that this same pathway leads to good mental health as well. The word Yoga, itself, stems from Sanskrit and means "union." This suggests that man's perfect role is that of being at one with the universe. In fact, peak physical and mental condition should be man's natural state.

In pursuing this role, one would ideally live without artificial foods and stormy emotions, and without becoming too reliant upon mechanical devices that sap the vitality. Yoga stresses this sensible approach to living as the only way that man can achieve his full potential.

Only natural foods should be consumed, according to these beliefs. This means that no food should be preserved, or altered, in preparation. This would eliminate all of the processed foodstuffs on the supermarket shelves.

All meats, vegetables and fruits should remain unchemicalized and unsprayed. While this type of pure food has grown scarce almost to the point of non-existence, there are farms now that cater to the newly awakening and growing concerns of Americans who want wholesome, natural foods.

These organic farms are on the increase, and do-it-yourself gardeners are learning that even a tiny area in a yard can produce a summer's supply of tasty vegetables.

As far as stormy emotions are concerned, they can deter man from being at one with the universe around him. Extremes of any emotion would suggest a need to examine the body and mind until the trouble's source is found. Yoga gets to the root of many mental distresses and discloses that physical malfunctioning can often create severe mental upheavals. By thoroughly exercising and flexing all body parts, better functioning of the glands that control the various mental states can be achieved. Many

NEW BODIES FOR OLD

toxins can be cleared from the system in this manner.

In addition, greater physical endurance comes about through Yoga exercises. As the movements are practiced, the body begins to know an ease of mobility that perhaps had disappeared with childhood.

It is a joyous feeling, this return of youthful comfort and ease. No matter what the age of the individual, a few simple Yoga exercises can bring a great sense of well-being. As one learns once again to use the legs for walking and the arms for moving and lifting, the overall health of the body will return. For the good results of moving one part of the body won't be limited to that specific area; the entire body, and the mind as well, will benefit.

Anyone Can Practice Yoga

Yoga imposes no strain on anyone who wishes to practice this discipline. Although there are many forms of Yoga, here we are concerned with Hatha Yoga only, which deals with physical well-being. Though the Hatha Yoga exercises are mainly concerned with the physical movements of the body, the mind profits also.

The body and mind profit from various "asanas", poses, or exercises (we use the words interchangeably) because of the fresh supply of oxygen that reaches previously neglected areas. So it is that alertness increases and a glow of life comes to our bodies with Yoga practices.

You *can* have that new body. You can know once again what it feels like to walk lightly, to sleep all night without awakening, to greet another with joy, and to approach each day with a deep sense of peace and contentment.

There is no magic involved in this re-creation. A minimum of fifteen minutes a day, less time than one takes for a coffee break, less time than one often spends on the telephone in casual conversation, and far less time than one would sit in a doctor's waiting room, will help restore you to glowing health.

Rediscover Your Body

Somewhere beneath the exterior appearance that might displease you or cause you discomfort or embarrassment, there is a sound body. Solid bone structure is there—basic and sound. The superfluous padding added over a period of time can be removed, toned, or reshaped. A flattened stomach that doesn't require a girdle can be achieved, and hips that fan out over a chair can be slimmed into proper shape.

With Yoga practices we can correct many figure faults, some of which can lead to actual physical distress if left unchecked. Legs can become shapely and pain-free with regular exercising. Thighs can be whittled down by carefully-selected movements that tighten and tone limbs padded with extra flesh.

Extra poundage that burdens the heart can be removed. Backs that have become stiffened with disuse can once again be called into supple play. And with all this reshaping and toning, an increase of self-awareness and self-appreciation can come about. With each advancement in the practice of Yoga, a desire for more benefits manifests itself. In this way, through an earnest striving to help one's body, a discipline is created that brings additional rewards.

Conscientiously applying oneself to a plan of self-improvement is not a simple matter of ego. Yoga teaches one to *know* his body, to *care* for his body in order to be free of needless physical woes.

All this cannot be done without a commitment, however. But it will be a wise commitment; a form of insurance of which you are the lifetime beneficiary. The decision to practice Yoga could become the most rewarding investment of time that you'll ever make.

The exercises in this book, if properly practiced, will return to you the body that perhaps you have lost to casual living and stress. For Hatha Yoga produces the inner calm that also creates outer beauty. Once you have known the deep peace of perfect calm and the grace of easy body movements, you will want to keep these exercises a part of your daily schedule.

The Need for Yoga

Yoga is not a religion, but an ancient discipline dating back over 3,000 years. Throughout these centuries, men and women concerned about their bodies have kept fit by performing these carefully planned exercises. In actual time, Yoga exercises require only minutes a day to create impressive changes in bodies prematurely aged by neglect and disuse.

Through the mild but sweeping movements, elasticity is regenerated within a body grown stiff from lack of movement. A gradual restoration of beauty and nimbleness begins to return after only a short period of practicing Yoga.

The body cannot feel beautiful or appear attractive when there is pain or discomfort felt in any area. The limbs are sometimes the first areas of the body to succumb to distresses brought about by faulty diet and lack of exercise. Leg cramps, weak ankles, and painful knees have crippling effects on body movement if left unchecked.

Such discomfort, in time, will reflect itself in little anxiety lines or wrinkles across the face. In this manner, malfunctioning of one part of the body writes its woes on others.

Yoga attacks these distresses at their source. Beginning with mild, gentle movements aimed at flexing the spine, graduated exercises manipulate every part of the body. The methodical exercises designed for various parts of the body help to remove stiffness and to restore strength.

As for calm, who does not have a need of this state? Who can afford to turn away from an undemanding discipline that revives a weary body and brings pleasure to everyday living?

The housewife, alone or with her children all day, requires tranquility in order to accomplish her tasks and reach her goals. The business man and woman must use their minds rather than their emotions to make decisions. The student must be free of debilitating passions in order to pursue his studies. And finally, the older person who finds his working days over, must know serenity if he is to enjoy his latter years.

Efficiency in any area of work is impaired by the slightest degree of irritability, annoyance or discomfort. With years spent in preparation for a life's work, it is an act of negligence to ignore simple physical needs. Essential and supple functioning of the body and mind is easily achieved by these exercises that bring increased awareness.

In practicing Yoga, both to control your emotions and to remold your figure, you will be involved with millions of others in a self-improvement program that does indeed bring both peace and beauty.

When we speak of true beauty, we are referring to an inner quality or an air of grace, instead of outward appearances. When we say of a structure, "That is a beautiful building," we do so usually because of good lines, careful construction, and a sense of rightness about the effect. We are not just referring to a coat of paint, a wall of windows, or some other outward decor. The building in question could be either a log cabin or a mansion. No matter what its type of construction, if it is unspoiled by artificial appurtenances, we can always find beauty in it.

When we say of a woman, "She is truly beautiful," it is because we sense a poise, an inner calm, and a beauty all of her own making. We are not referring to youth alone, or a smoothly made-up face, a labored coiffure, or elegant clothes.

We usually refer to this facade as smart, chic, or glamorous—never beautiful.

While the outward appearances are a part of the overall whole, if the inner qualities of calm and grace are not present, there is a jarring element. We consider it a betrayal to our senses when we see a pretty woman sitting awkwardly in her chair, standing with poor posture, or walking in an ungainly fashion.

To be able to discern beauty in its true form enables us to work toward these qualities within ourselves. With Yoga practices, we can correct many figure faults, some of which might lead to actual physical distress if left unchecked.

Sagging waistlines can be firmed, tautened, and made smaller. It is a common occurrence to lose several inches from the waist after practicing Yoga exercises. In fact, tone comes to all parts of the body with Yoga. A neck that has developed loose, hanging folds of flesh can be greatly improved and strengthened. Flabby underarms become youthful and attractive when the proper movements are practiced.

Hips and thighs can be reduced to correct proportions. Weak ankles can be made strong. Stooped shoulders resulting from poor posture can be corrected, and all other areas of the body can profit by simple but thorough Yoga.

The Yoga method is simplicity itself; there are no outside "helps" necessary. As a matter of fact, one doesn't even have to leave home to follow the pathway to beauty and good health that this discipline offers. Improvement can be had with no more equipment than one's own body, the set of Yoga exercises, and a determination to rescue oneself.

And this is what Hatha Yoga is all about. Its aim is to get you to flexing parts of the body that otherwise will grow lethargic and weak in disuse.

Otherwise when that debilitating action commences, you will begin to wonder where that marvelous energy of youth disappeared, and what happened to the legs that once carried you so confidently through your days. Or why you no longer can bend with ease, or reach above you without the almost unbearable reminder that you are no longer in full, comfortable control of your own body.

You Are As Young As Your Spine Is Flexible

It can come as a shock that you are no longer in command of the machine that was born in grace and beauty to bend, reach, pull, push, or stretch for you. It is a depressing fact that neglected muscles rebel, joints ache, and bones resist if you have ignored your body.

The physical exercises of Yoga help one to gain control over one's body again, to increase self-confidence, and to overcome fatigue and tension. This practice can also tighten the body into a beautiful physical shape even as it serves to calm the mind.

When you have an aching back, you cannot possibly pursue your day's work with the same spirit that you would know if your back were without pain. When you have a headache, your immediate desire is to turn aside from whatever demanding task is at hand and find some place to rest the throbbing temples.

The strongest desire within us at such a time is to find a place of complete quiet. And yet, if our bodies were in good condition, it is there we would find this state of constant tranquility. The body should be the temple of all serenity; a place to which one can retreat in peace when outside forces grow strident and one needs to gain composure and a refreshed mental attitude.

One might wonder: How can such a simple practice as Yoga provide all these things? To answer that question, we've only to remember that life in its most essential form is not complicated. It is civilization's demanding customs and barbarous activities that have made it so. When we shed our superficially created methods of living, we are left with very simple habits.

Eliminate the second car in your family and someone would have to walk somewhere some of the time. Eliminate all cars and the whole family would be forced to walk and, inconvenience notwithstanding, every one would probably benefit greatly from the resulting body movements.

And it is this that Yoga stresses. Move your body. Bend, reach, stretch, roll, stoop, flex, and shrug. Use your body. Use it wisely and sensibly and do not permit equipment (electric appliances) and machinery (automobiles, outboard motors, etc.) to take over all the beneficial body movements. The body that is vibrant from use is the body that is really alive, and one that requires no artificial stimulation from coffee, pills, or cigarettes.

Natural stimulation quickens blood circulation to the point that more nourishment and fresh oxygen are carried to previously neglected areas of the body. This in turn creates a person who, because of being more alive, is more creative and content.

Your body is your most prized possession. Dependent upon your state of health and in accordance with what you do to your body, you can accomplish any goal. With a healthy mind and body, you can realize success more easily in whatever you want to do. Such success is not possible if you permit the stresses of the time to reach you because you have ignored the needs of your body.

According to Dr. Hans Selye, director of the University of Montreal's Institute of Experimental Medicine and Surgery, an automobile doesn't suddenly stop running because of old age. Rather, it stops because of failure of some specific part that has worn out. Relating that to people under continuous stress that is either physical or mental, some vital part of the body gives way, leading to a variety of illnesses, and eventually, to death.

The Viennese doctor's experiments with rats brought glaring proof of the destructive effects of stress. Whether the stress introduced to the rats was from fatigue, frustration, anger, or any one of a dozen other emotions, the result was the same: Internal wreckage on a gigantic scale took place. Glandular disturbances were extreme; blood pressure rose and ulcers developed.

Since humans are subject to similar stresses, one can understand their reactions would be comparable. And the sources of stress increase daily in our own rushed, hectic, anxiety-ridden world. Obviously, if we cannot change the conditions that produce death-dealing stresses, then we must learn to avoid the resultant damage.

Yoga can teach one to cope with any and all situations that involve the emotions to the point that even under harrowing circumstances one remains serene. The Yoga method of achieving calm is so effective that you can leave your office, place of business or home no more ruffled after decision making than had you gone for a solitary walk down a peaceful country lane.

In addition to regular Yoga practices, deep breathing exercises will help to bring this about. The deep breathing technique is practiced with all Yoga postures, and can completely remove tensions and the effects of strain from your life. Mastering deep breathing and employing it in any unnerving situation can also help one to avoid an emotional outburst—still another factor in body breakdown.

We know that irritability or anger never improved a situation. On the contrary, the picture changes in proportion to our own handling of it, and how well we are able to quiet our distressed emotions. It is these passions which etch themselves across our face, or show themselves elsewhere on our body.

Abuse and disuse of the body ravage both from within and without. There can not possibly be real inner peace and beauty until control is brought to all parts of the body.

Discover Your Body

Genuine beauty is composed of many qualities. It is the fluidity of movement and the erectness of carriage that shows a person is at ease with his own body and proud of its appearance. Whether the person is tall, short, thin or heavy boned, if he holds himself erectly, one's immediate response is a sense of pleasure in that person's control of his body.

Another quality of beauty is composure. A nervous, fidgety person is distracting to watch, and causes uneasiness among those around him. Lack of composure detracts mightily from any physical attribute. Inner calm can cover the body and bring serenity to uneven features.

There are progressive changes that take place in both the physical and mental condition with steady day-to-day exercises. Since all bodies are unique and therefore will respond differently, each participant will take from Yoga and benefit from it according to his need. For some, advances will be made at an incredible rate. For others, a plateau of performance may be reached and a levelling off of benefits may set in.

At times there may even be a resistance to improvement. This is especially true of the unusually neglected body and the body that has already stiffened with disuse. But one shouldn't be discouraged. With faithful practice and a determined attitude to reach higher and higher until the beautiful body is attained, another level will be reached, and dramatic improvement will eventually come.

Within the body is a reservoir of untapped energy. This has to be acknowledged because in times of stress, or at moments of great need, unbelievable strength can be called forth to meet emergency demands. Because so little is known or understood about this latent force that needs only tending or developing to supply sufficient energy for one's entire life, we usually accept daily fatigue as an ungovernable fact.

NEW BODIES FOR OLD

The truth of the matter is that with proper care to the body, one never need be exhausted or greatly fatigued. Increased vitality comes with understanding and promoting the proper functioning of the body. Obviously one cannot have this super-power if one neglects or abuses one's body. At the same time, one cannot expect to rely upon an everlasting source of strength if the body isn't properly exercised and kept elastic.

Yoga is unique in its ability to nurture the body and to coax it to its finest performance. And it is this discipline, working to bring out the best in you, that can also help you not only to be healthy and alert in your youthful years, but also to meet and greet your middle and older years with vibrant health.

When youth is upon one, sickness is comparatively easy to overcome. But if the older body has been neglected, the organs abused, and the body tone allowed to grow flaccid, then later illnesses have a much greater striking force.

What use, then, are extra years, if one is stricken with debilitating diseases and collapse of first one organ and then another?

Yoga concerns itself not only with the outer person but with the inner organs that carry the burden of our life processes. Not one Yoga movement is designed without some benefit to the inner workings of the body. A movement of the leg may pull also on the stomach area and bring tone even as the leg is being flexed in order to develop tone there. A roll of the head will bring ease of activity to the spine that has stiffened from lack of use.

The bending of the waist will pull on the rib cage and relax the back muscles. Even a complete relaxation posture, when one is lying supine without moving any part of the body, brings a release to tightly held muscles, and soothes nerves that have been tautened by stress or other wear.

Curative powers are unleashed when accumulated toxins are forced from the body by its own natural defenses. But in order to build a fortress of the physique and mentality; in order to create a citadel of strength to meet the growing demands of a frantic society, it is necessary to treat oneself as a whole, and to work not on just one part of the body, or of the mind.

Yoga believes that proper treatment of the body can insure happy and rewarding years ahead. Such youthful characteristics as an agile body and an alert mind can be enjoyed beyond those years that we measure and set aside as belonging to a certain age group. The stiffened, unattractive movements we associate with great age need not be experienced by anyone who cares to renew or remake or restore his body.

The results of such concern produce the men and women who can continue to dance across a stage well into their senior years, or to pursue a profession that brings them pleasure long after more sedentary people have retired from life.

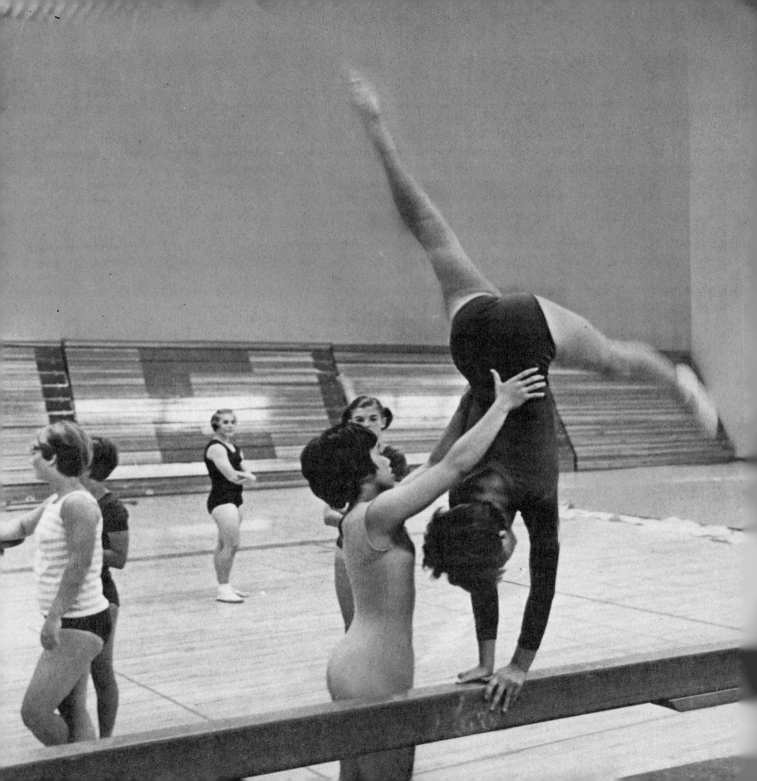

CHAPTER TWO - A SUPPLE SPINE IS THE KEY

There are a few simple rules to observe as you begin to practice Yoga exercises. These rules pertain to the comfort and protection of your body, and you will benefit by observing them.

Food should not be taken for two hours before practicing Yoga. This is in order to avoid discomfort and interruption of the processes of digestion.

You will want to be attired in comfortable clothing which will permit you to move about freely. Belts and shoes must be removed, and nothing of a restricting nature should be worn. Leotards are excellent for exercising. Or you could wear a one-piece playsuit, gym shorts, or sweat pants. The idea is to permit your body the complete freedom of movement necessary for acquiring confidence in your body postures.

Perform your exercises on a mat, quilt, blanket, or carpeted floor, in order to have protection for your body as you move it in these unaccustomed poses. There is much greater ease of movement this way.

Slowness of performance is always essential in Yoga exercises. We are trying to slow our bodies down in order to help control the nervous tension that can arise from hasty movements and compulsive action. This is a very important part of Yoga. Nothing is done swiftly. It is far better to perform only half the number of exercises at a leisurely pace than to double the number and do them at a fast clip.

One should never rush to perfect any movement. When you see an illustration of a Yoga posture, you are seeing the ultimate goal rather than the beginning of the performance. Remember, a teacher or advanced student who can perform the postures with ease also had to be a beginner once, and was not always so agile. So do not compare your first movements with those of final accomplishment.

And never compare your body to that of another. This is completely unfair, for no two bodies are alike. One person's area of strength may be another's weakness, and vice versa. You will find many exercises that you consider impossible, but others that seem to come easily. This is true of everyone, for we all have used our bodies in different ways. Yoga's purpose is to bring one and all to good form and litheness.

Remember that the inclination to rush and try to make up for lost time, once you have started a regular pattern of exercising, must be avoided. Do not try to gain an alacrity of movement within a short time. This will come with daily practice, and you will benefit all the more from your efforts if you perform in moderation.

To begin our exercises, we want to aim for an all encompassing limbering movement. This means we want to work on the overall body without limiting ourselves to one specific part of the anatomy. Yoga treats the body as a whole, and works in an orderly manner to build up the general flexibility of the entire body.

While the temptation may be to dash through the preliminary exercises in search of specific ones, this is not the practical way. For these exercises have been scientifically planned, with one leading into the other as the general tone of the body is improved. In order to produce the greatest benefits, the exercises should be practiced in the prescribed order.

The spine is usually in the greatest need of limbering since it controls many functions of the mind and body. Real health and ease of movement can come only if there is complete suppleness of the spine.

When a child tumbles joyously and fearlessly, it is because he feels no restriction from this area. His spinal column is as flexible as his hand, therefore he uses it with the same degree of ease. If the child falls, the supple spine bends with him, and in this manner he avoids serious injury.

But as we grow older we lose this marvelous flexibility. We are children no longer, and so we feel we should no longer tumble and bend. We are rushed into another form of living that requires long hours in a seated position while we prepare for "life". The less we move about with spontaneous and frequent use of our body, the more rigid and stiff the spinal column grows. From lack of use, it will eventually resist even the slightest bending movements, and the growing discomfort we experience from trying to curve a rigid spine tells us to avoid further movements that might intensify this distress.

So we begin down the road that leads to premature aging. For it is well known that a person who remains active throughout his life also retains a more youthful appearance, and certainly, a more flexible and therefore youthful spine.

Without a flexible spine, you cannot successfully perform even the most elementary movements. A supple spine brings other benefits: good carriage, a graceful walk, and a more attractive appearance.

Many women who complain of a too-small bust would actually show their body at its loveliest and shapeliest if they would simply practice good posture. And good posture depends upon a supple spine.

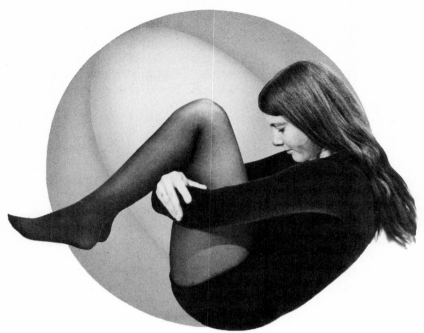

Rock and Roll

To limber up the spine, we begin by practicing the Rock and Roll movement. Truly one of the most satisfying motions in which we can indulge, the Rock and Roll curves our body into a ball and helps to add the desired suppleness to our spine.

Gather yourself into a rounded position as you sit on the floor. Bring your knees up under your chin and tuck your head down to meet the tops of your knees. Try to visualize your body rounded into the shape of a large ball. Grasp the under thighs with the arms loosely interlaced, if possible. If this position of the arms is not possible, then allow the hands to hold the legs separately.

A second position that some may prefer is that of clasping the outside of the legs with the arms, rather than clasping the thighs. Try both methods and determine which one is more comfortable for you.

With the head bent downward toward the knees, slowly roll backward onto the floor. Remember to keep the back as rounded as possible, or you will find yourself flat on the floor without the momentum needed to return to a sitting position.

Keep the body in motion as you roll backward once again. Visualize a rocking chair and adopt the same movement.

Practice this movement several times. If you find that you don't roll well, or that you cannot roll forward into a sitting position once you have rolled backward onto the floor, don't be discouraged. This will remedy itself with practice. And the rewards for your efforts will be many. With daily practice of the Rock and Roll, the spine begins to limber up and tension and strain that gather at the top of the vertebrae begin to disappear. There is also an increased blood circulation throughout the body.

Many people find the Rock and Roll the ideal way to begin a day. Performed each morning, it can send you forth with a lighter step and a sense of readiness to meet the day because of the increased stimulation to the body.

Not only does the Rock and Roll limber the spine and remove stiffness from that area; it is also useful in getting to sleep. Because tension seems to gather first at the top of the spine, when we gently massage this area by the delicious rocking motion, we are soothing the distressed area and relaxing the muscles.

The Rock and Roll should always begin your daily exercise, no matter what time of the day you practice. Whether you choose the early morning or late evening to do your exercises, try to be consistent. If you decide to practice Yoga before retiring each night, try to keep the same hour if possible. In this way you will be more inclined to observe the practice as a way of life, rather than following a hit-or-miss schedule that has to adjust itself to your other needs.

Deep Breathing

In order to breathe correctly when we are doing Yoga exercises, it is necessary to understand the structure and purpose of the lungs.

Deep breathing is a spontaneous way of taking in oxygen as we sleep, and it is the natural way of breathing for babies and animals. But we short-cut this practice along with many other health practices as we mature.

The pear-shaped lung organ draws in oxygen and sends it on to the bloodstream. By this action, the blood is bathed and purified. In the process the cells of the body are repaired and restored. It is through the deep breathing techniques that the vital life force of oxygen is carried along to previously neglected areas.

In turn, this stimulates and revives circulation and brings about a sense of rejuvenation to all parts of the body.

Wastes are removed from the body by exhaling. The quantity of wastes removed by this purifying gaseous exchange of oxygen for carbon dioxide is determined by our method of breathing. It is therefore logical that shallow breathing will not bring about the cleansing of the bloodstream that deep breathing will.

In the beginning, deep breathing is to be practiced only during the Yoga exercises, and at no other time. Upon completion of the exercises, breathing should return to normal. As you master the technique of deep breathing, you will more and more employ this method of taking in an extra quantity of oxygen to relieve tension as it begins to build up in your body.

Later, you will want to deep breathe at different times of the day when you feel a sense of fatigue. At no time will it completely supplant normal breathing. Several deep breaths, taken at varying times, will supply you with the fresh oxygen supply needed to calm, or stimulate, your body at any given time. So beneficial is this deep breathing that it can be substituted for the usual cup of coffee, cigarette, or even stronger stimulant.

Causes of Poor Breathing Habits

Poor posture helps to bring about reduced oxygen intake. Often as we busy ourselves acquiring knowledge, we neglect our bodies and lose the physical abandon we knew as children. The result is invariably detrimental. While it is possible to be of a scholarly nature and in good health at the same time, generally speaking, we perform our mental occupations in a restricted pose.

Observe a young high school or college student as he involves himself in his studies. Nine times out of ten he will hollow his chest, round his shoulders, and bend forward, absorbed in his book. His arms are usually drawn tightly toward the chest while the forehead leans heavily on his hands.

He takes short, shallow breaths, not really capable of supplying the body, much less the brain, with the much-needed oxygen required for absorbing and retaining knowledge. How much of what he is struggling to learn will stay with him? With a mind that is fuzzy and dull from oxygen starvation, his efforts are greatly hampered.

Study would be far more productive if the student were in a well-ventilated area, sitting upright in a comfortably firm chair with a relaxed body and a well-nourished brain that could readily absorb all that was fed it.

But this is not the way of our civilized society, and it is definitely not the way of most individuals who work under pressure. Only conscious effort can change the debilitating habit of shallow breathing that deprives the body of life-giving and life-restoring oxygen.

Deep breathing methods, as taught in Hatha Yoga, are completely different from those we learned as children. Generally speaking, when one untutored in the correct deep breathing exercises steps out into a crisp, fresh day and attempts to take in a deep breath, he throws out his chest, pulls in his stomach, and attempts to deep breathe.

The air intake in this case is strictly limited, and really supplies a small amount of oxygen compared to what the body requires.

In Yoga deep breathing, oxygen is taken in through the nostrils with the mouth closed. The oxygen is consciously directed to the lowest reaches of the abdomen without movement from the chest area.

Without proper attention to oxygen intake, the aging process is hurried along. This can be easily understood when we realize that the living cells which compose our body receive their life-sustaining nutrition and oxygen through the bloodstream, and that the bloodstream itself depends on oxygen intake. The constant breakdown and repair of cells that must go on as long as there is life, is dependent on the oxygen we breathe so casually. When the oxygen supply is limited, the maintenance of the entire body suffers, and the consequence is early aging.

To begin the practice of deep breathing, think of yourself as an empty pitcher. You are going to fill this empty pitcher with oxygen the same way you would fill it with water; from the bottom up. As you inhale oxygen through the nose, with the mouth closed, your abdominal muscles slowly lift up the lower stomach region, or bottom of the pitcher.

After the bottom region is filled, the middle region is next, and then, slowly, the upper or chest region is filled with air.

Keep the chest area motionless, let the diaphragm do the work. This is very important, and usually requires practice to bring about the coordination needed.

Only the abdominal muscles should expand as air is taken in. In this method of breathing, one takes in the greatest amount of oxygen with the least amount of effort. For exhaling, release the air slowly from the chest area first, then the middle area and finally the lower region, again using only the abdominal muscles.

This exercise is to be practiced slowly, in a completely relaxed position as you lie flat on the floor in a well-ventilated room. Never practice deep breathing in a close atmosphere. Of course, you would not practice it, either, in a smoked-filled room, on a crowded bus, or any area where the oxygen intake would be of dubious, or even harmful, value. The purpose of the deep breathing is to take in oxygen, and you would not be helped by breathing in stale air.

Practice no more than three times the first day. After that, you will use the deep breathing with each of your exercises. Excessive deep breathing may bring on dizziness because you are unaccustomed to this great amount of oxygen coming into your body. In time you will learn to apply this technique to various situations in order to prevent tension build-up in your body. But in the beginning, practice with restraint.

Sitting Postures

After we have learned to deep breathe, we must learn how to get into the postures that lead us into a state of health. There are six methods of sitting that will help guide us as we move on to our beneficial exercises. The six positions lead the body slowly and undemandingly into the first movements to elasticize stiffened joints and to gain back a measure of the freedom one had as a child.

As you make progress with other Yoga movements, you will come to look upon these original six methods of sitting as very mild and exceedingly simple. But to enter a program of reclaiming the body, it is essential that the program have an easy entrance, and that exercises or positions be of a mild nature.

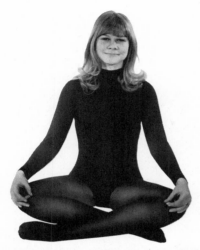

The Easy Pose

This basic sitting position may not be easy for all, but it is the beginning of Yogic positions. In order to get into this posture, sit on the floor and cross your legs tailor-fashion in the manner in which we sat as children. The heels of both feet rest against the inner thigh of the other leg.

Keep the spine straight. This in turn will help to strengthen the back muscles and to improve your posture. Remain in this position only as long as you are comfortable. But do not miss a single day in its practice, for it is the unfailing, day-in and day-out repetition that will help to stretch and strengthen the unused and taut muscles of this part of the body.

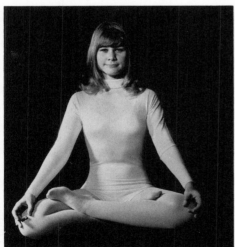

Perfect Pose

In a sitting position on the floor, place the heel of the left leg on the upper, inner thigh of the right leg, as close in to the crotch as possible, with the sole turned upwards, while the right foot presses against the left thigh. The knees should touch the floor.

Do not force the legs to bend, and do not sustain the position if it is uncomfortable. Work gradually toward perfecting this pose, and allow as much time as is needed. Daily practice will help you ease into this position.

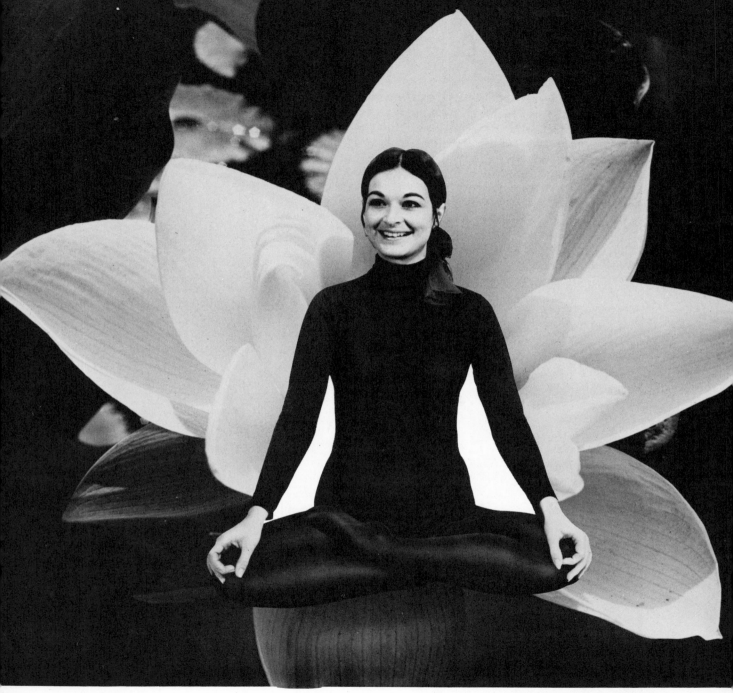

A SUPPLE SPINE IS THE KEY

Lotus Pose

In a seated position on the floor, place the right foot on the left thigh, pulling the right ankle closely in toward the groin. Lift the left leg and cross it over the right leg to place the left foot onto the right thigh.

Both knees should touch the floor. If the position is difficult, work toward this pose gradually by learning to bounce your knees. This applies to the first two sitting positions, also.

To gain flexibility by bouncing, place the right leg straight out in front of you, and put the foot of the left leg flat against the inner thigh. With your hand placed palm downward on the bent knee, gently bounce the knee to the floor, or as close to it as is comfortably possible. Do this several times and then change leg positions and repeat the movement with the right knee.

When continued practice limbers the muscles and permits the knee to touch the floor, raise the foot to rest on top of the thigh and bounce the knee from the higher position. Use this bouncing exercise for both knees, if needed.

In time this bouncing action will limber the thigh and knee areas enough to permit all three of the previously mentioned sitting positions.

Few people can perform the lotus position without practice, so don't be discouraged if you must prepare for the sitting positions by bouncing the knee for a long period of time in order to gain the needed flexibility. Our Western world devised the chair, and in using this supportive structure, we avoid the necessary stretching of the muscles of our legs. This in turn creates a weakness and inelasticity in that area. The people in the East who can sit for hours with their legs crossed in tailor fashion are not great exponents of the chair.

While we wouldn't want to sit on the floor all the time, and though this is not our goal, nevertheless, we do want our bodies to be flexible and pain free. And in acquiring leg muscles that are not too taut to permit easy use of them, we are working toward that comfortable condition.

The lotus position, itself, is also called the locked position. This is because once in the lotus position, one can neither roll or fall backward or forward. This is an important factor in meditation, when complete security of the body position is sought while the mind rests or moves beyond thoughts pertaining to the physical.

While the lotus position is a pretty pose, and is a stylized picture of all Yoga, it is not necessarily more important than any other position called for in the practice of Yoga. In fact, there are a great many positions of much greater strengthening value in that they call for more coordinated movement of more parts of the body.

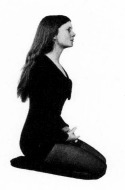

Kneeling Position

With the knees bent to the floor, sit with the buttocks on the heels. Keep the back straight. Arms can hang easily by the side, or be lightly folded in the lap area. Maintain this position for a few minutes to accustom the legs to the pull. With steady practice this pose becomes very easily managed. In the beginning however, some may find it a bit awkward.

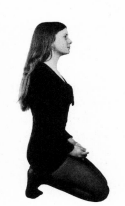

Kneeling With the Toes Tucked Under

Sit in the kneeling position described above, but this time tuck the toes under the feet in an opposite direction, pointed frontwards, so that along with the knees, they are supporting the body.

You won't be able to hold this position very long in the beginning. It is an unaccustomed position, but one that is very beneficial in its strengthening of the toes. Gradually, as the toes gain in strength the discomfort will disappear.

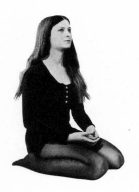

Kneeling Sitting Between the Legs

With the knees bent to the floor, spread them enough to permit the lowering of the hips between them. Lower the hips slowly until they come to rest between the legs and the buttocks have touched the floor. The toes are in a normal position here.

If you find yourself unable to lower the buttocks to the floor, reach behind with your hands and grasp your up-turned heels. Gently rock yourself up and down, being careful not to force movement where it is uncomfortable. Rock hips in this vertical position until they have gained the need flexibility for lowering themselves to the floor.

A SUPPLE SPINE IS THE KEY

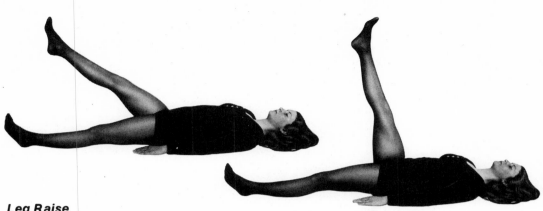

Leg Raise

Lie flat on the floor with your hands alongside your body. Breathe deeply and raise one leg as high as you comfortably can, aiming at a 90 degree angle, or right angle to the body.

Keep the knees straight; both the one on the floor and the raised one. Exhale slowly and lower the leg. Do not force the leg upward beyond a point of comfort. If you cannot reach a 90 degree angle without bending your knee, go only as far as the knee remains comfortably unbent.

Relax.

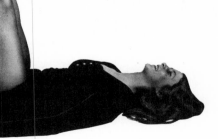

Repeat this exercise with the right leg, remembering to deep breathe. Relax. Then raise both legs at one time, and slowly lower them. Do not permit the legs to fall to the floor. Your movements must be controlled at all times. Try to hold the back rather firmly to the floor during the leg raise. This is especially important during the lowering of both legs at one time.

Work at this daily, and in time you will be able to achieve the 90 degree angle of the legs.

LOOK YOUNGER - LOOK PRETTIER

Reversed Leg Raise

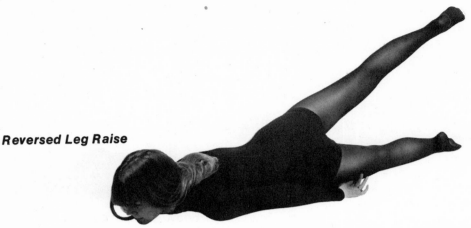

Lie flat on the stomach. Place your arms alongside your body. Breathe deeply and raise one leg as high behind you as you comfortably can. Your head should be supported by the chin or forehead.

Keep both the knee that is remaining on the floor and the one that is being lifted straight. Keep the muscles relaxed. Exhale and slowly bring the leg down. Relax. Inhale and raise the other leg in the same manner, keeping the muscles relaxed. Exhale and slowly bring the leg down. Relax.

Do not strain or force the leg back and upward beyond a point of comfort. In the beginning you may be able to lift the leg only a few inches or a foot. But there is no deadline on Yoga practices to reach a greater height. Let your comfort dictate the height your leg will reach.

Do not raise both legs at one time.

EXERCISES AND BENEFITS IN CHAPTER 2

Rock and Roll—This rounded position is used to limber the body and prepare it for various positions. It is also helpful in reducing tension, and is sleep conducive if practiced before retiring. The gentle rolling movements are a form of massage for the vertebrae and are helpful in relaxing the area which tends to tighten from anxiety build-up.

Many people find they can start a day more agreeably by doing a few rock and rolls immediately upon arising. Because of the stepped up circulation produced by the rocking, there is a quicker awakening and a loss of early morning sluggishness.

Easy Pose—This is the first seated position. In this posture, the legs receive a gentle and mild stretching that is stimulating and helpful in activating long-unused muscles and ligaments.

Perfect Pose—This position begins the stretching of the thighs and lower back, necessary in order to proceed more comfortably to other positions.

Lotus Pose—The knee joints and ankles receive beneficial stretching which creates a greater sense of ease. Once learned, the lotus is the position used for meditation because of its security and comfort.

Kneeling Posture—The kneejoints and the thighs receive a gentle stretching, and the straightened back is a reminder of good posture.

Kneeling With the Toes Tucked Under—The same benefits are received as in the above exercise, with the added advantage of strengthening the toes, which in turn creates better balance. Poise is much assisted by practicing this position. Better balance enables us to walk up and down stairs with greater ease and to turn quickly.

Kneeling Sitting Between the Legs—This is an excellent exercise for strengthening the leg muscles. It is also of great value in moving the hips and flexing the hip joints.

Leg Raise—This exercise massages the organs in the abdomen and firms its muscles. It is considered one of the best exercises for a flabby abdomen, and it is also an aid to good posture. With daily practice of the leg raise, there is increased tone to the peristalsis action of the intestines. The muscle corset that girds the abdomen is toned and strengthened by this exercise to the point that one can usually, in time, give up the wearing of corsets and girdles for support.

Reversed Leg Raise—The back muscles benefit in this opposite stretch to the leg raise. Auxiliary muscles are strengthened, which in turn may increase sexual abilities.

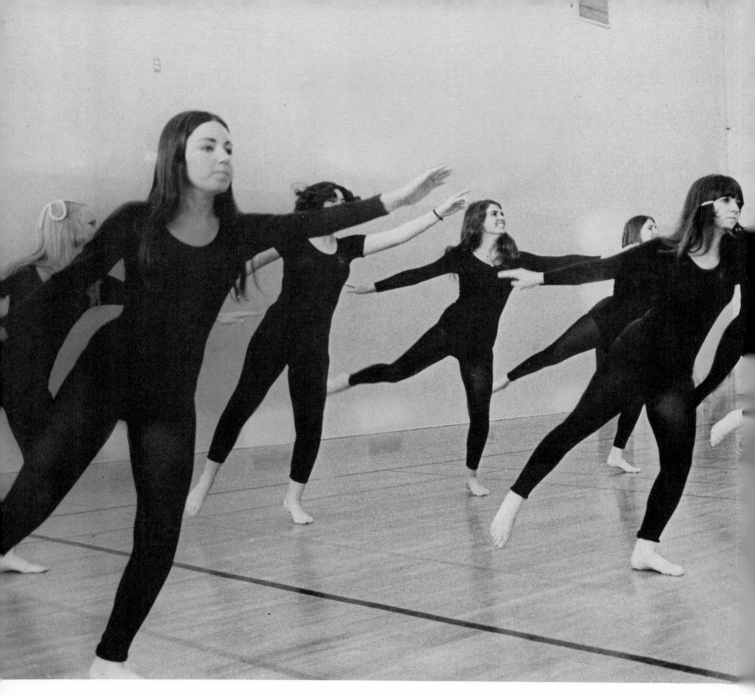

YOGA REWARDS THOSE WHO PERSEVERE

CHAPTER THREE — YOGA REWARDS THOSE WHO PERSEVERE

By now you have had time to try the various positions and exercises, and your body is beginning to loosen up a bit. There may be a little discomfort in certain areas because of the unaccustomed activity. However, remember that in no exercise are you to perform to the point that you feel any pain.

Keep in mind that Yoga stresses slow mastery over your body, as the more effective and safer way. You can only do damage by rushing into any physical movement. Work slowly, not striving for any perfection of performance, but rather for a sense of comfort in the working of your body.

You must realize that you are moving, stretching, and therefore restoring to normal elasticity areas of your body that have not known this activity in many years, perhaps. Because of this, slight discomfort may come about. To avoid such aches, you might choose to abstain from those particular exercises for a day or two, before returning to them. Usually one or two days away from the exercise is enough to cause any discomfort to disappear. Then you are free to commence again, very gently and without too much vigor.

A body that has been without daily exercise for a period of time is naturally going to rebel when introduced to greater movement than usual. It takes an effort to create anything of beauty and usefulness. We cannot expect that the monumental accomplishment of changing an aging or distressed body can come about without some sense of dedication.

It seems easier, perhaps, to accept a pain and say, "I have a weak back and have to be careful." Or, "I have arthritis and cannot move my limbs very much." But all the more reason to pay attention to the body's need for a definite plan of exercise. Obviously ailments aren't going to disappear by leading a sedentary life. The path of acceptance, indifference, and smugness will cut a life short, make it miserable, and will deny one the joys of being really alive and well.

Let me cite some specific examples of recent date from my own students, who have realized tremendous benefits from the study and practice of the physical exercises of Yoga—benefits which border on the miraculous in their effectiveness.

Jackie came into class after losing twenty pounds of excess weight; a tall, striking brunette, but her body was in need of toning. She had other problems, too, she said, but the first thing she wanted to accomplish with Yoga was to tighten the loose flesh on her body which had resulted from her admirable loss of weight.

She really labored in the beginning, trying to learn to roll in a ball position; to gather her resisting body and command it to move. Others in the class learned to roll. Jackie flipped off her mat sideways. But she persisted with her efforts and was rewarded with a developing suppleness.

However, she insisted that she really felt no better for all her efforts, after some weeks. She was told that different people respond and react to Yoga in entirely different ways. There are those who, upon beginning the exercises, burst forth as changed people once the blood circulation has aroused their lethargic bodies. Others go for a much longer period of time before a change will manifest itself.

But the change will come. Of that there is no doubt. Daily practice will bring it about.

With Jackie's determination to rescue her body she eventually found the rewards she sought. Halfway through the course she burst into the studio in exuberant spirits.

The previous week she had discovered that the painful menstrual periods she had known for eighteen years had disappeared. There were other benefits, too. She was sleeping better, and had seemed to acquire a tremendous amount of energy.

Each following week Jackie would inform the class of some marvelous change in her body or disposition. And the class listened and believed, for most of them had experienced similar benefits at an earlier date.

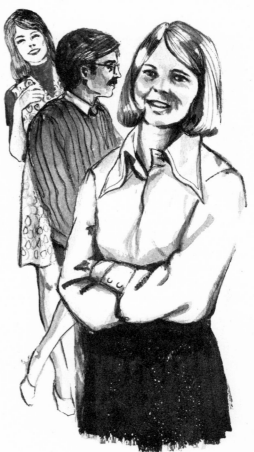

Jackie, Ron and Sharon

There were others who benefitted in additional ways. Ron had a demanding job in the map department of his company. Most of his day was spent hunched over finely drawn lines that he followed with a magnifying glass. By the end of the day he was exhausted, cross, headachy, and restless.

His wife had been practicing Yoga for some time and eventually she persuaded him to join a class in order to learn to relax. He wasn't difficult to convince, for he was aware that his wife's improved spirit and health had commenced with Yoga exercises.

Within a matter of a few weeks after starting Yoga himself, Ron noticed that his headaches had disappeared, his eyes were not burning at the end of the day, and he was able to unwind early in the evening. The neck rolls had once again done their incredible work.

The increased blood circulation to the ophthalmic nerves had given him better vision. Later, when he went to his optometrist for a checkup, he found that he did not have to have the usual lens change because his eyes were stronger.

Sharon was a pretty girl who looked as though she had just been insulted by the world. Lithe of body and trim of line, she had turned to Yoga, she said, because she had so many free evenings and nothing of importance to do.

That was the only reason?

Well, she did feel pretty grumpy most of the time. If someone said something to her, she always seemed to look for hidden barbs, for she knew she didn't have the best disposition. But then, why should she? With other people being so critical of her, it was natural to respond in kind, wasn't it?

Even while justifying her perhaps unpleasant disposition, Sharon was seeking help, for she was an intelligent person and she knew that she was not getting much out of her life. So she was here, and where was all that serenity and peacefulness she had heard about in relation to Yoga?

It didn't take long with Sharon. She said it was the Waking Up exercises that did it. They were, she said, an open door to a good day. Apparently Sharon had never awakened in a pleasant manner. She slept each morning until the last moment and then she threw herself into preparations for the day that started her off with built up tensions that increased with every hour.

Practicing the exercises that help one respond pleasantly to a new day, Sharon no longer snapped at the first person who spoke to her each morning. Nor the second or third or fourth. She lost her irritability and gained a relaxed attitude not possible with her previous method of brutally awakening her body each day.

You might say that a simple Yoga posture known as the Tree helped to hold a marriage together. Jocelyn's husband was a sailor in his spare time. Every weekend found him headed for the shore and his boat. Jocelyn encouraged this for her husband worked in a very high-pressure job. She felt he needed the relaxed weekends to help him untangle from his demanding position.

But Jocelyn was a landlubber and the sight of a wave in motion turned her green. She could not in any comfort board her husband's boat and this meant that most of his free and relaxed moments were spent away from her.

Jocelyn joined the Yoga class to have something to do when her husband was away. But when she heard of the benefits of the Tree, she began to practice it relentlessly. At any odd moment she would shuck her shoes and assume the position suggestive of a tree in its upright stance. The motion sickness with which she had been afflicted gradually subsided until Jocelyn could join her husband on his boat with a great measure of comfort. Now they both head for the shore together.

Begin each lesson with the Rocking exercise. As your body rolls backward, remember to check for deep breathing. By now you will be able to coordinate the deep breathing and the exercises better. Try for the coordination of inhaling as you roll backward, and exhaling as you return frontward. Aim for slow and steady movements, and try to avoid hurried thrusts as you roll backward.

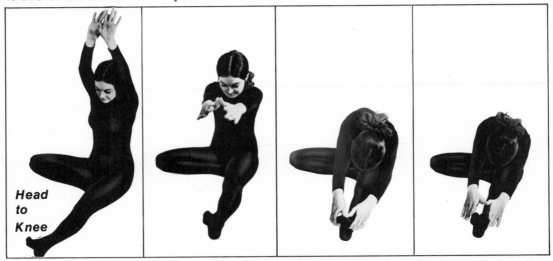

Head to Knee

Sit in an upright position with the spine held erectly. Place both legs in a straight line before you. Pull in the right leg and place the foot of that leg against the inner thigh of the left leg which remains in a straight position before you.

Inhale deeply and raise both arms overhead, with the elbows unbent. Exhale and lower the arms in a straight line before you. Slowly reach for the feet, with the head tucked toward the knee.

YOGA REWARDS THOSE WHO PERSEVERE

Do not rock the body back and forth in an attempt to reach the feet with your hands. Go only as far as you can without pushing the body or forcing the spine to bend beyond comfort.

Now repeat the exercise with the left leg pulled in, remembering to deep breathe. Relax again, and then place both legs before you in a straight line. Now reach for both feet with your hands, lowering your head toward your knees while you deep breathe in and out.

Hold this position for a few moments before slowly returning to an upright seated position. Do not strain forward in an attempt to reach the ultimate position of this pose. At all times, the goal must remain an individual one. If your fingers can reach no further than your knees without discomfort, then be satisfied for the day with that stretch. Each succeeding day's practice will bring more litheness to your spine, more circulation within your body. These are the day to day goals. The final goal of the pictured exercise will come by itself, if this slow, methodical approach is used.

Sudden and forced stretching of the spine can be damaging. At no time is the body to be pushed beyond its comfortable ability.

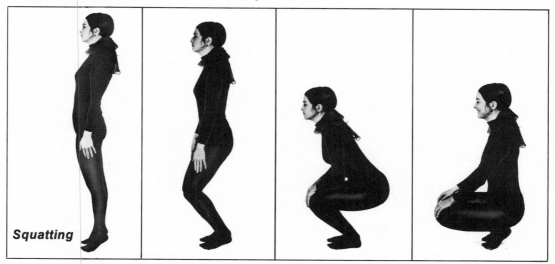

Squatting

In a standing position with the spine held straight, take a deep breath and go up on your toes. With the arms hanging easily by your sides, exhale as you bend your knees while lowering the body until the buttocks are resting on the heels. The arms will rest lightly on a line with the thighs while the hands rest against the knees.

Remain in this position for only a few moments in the beginning. Gradually work up to two or three minutes for additional strengthening of the thighs.

LOOK YOUNGER - LOOK PRETTIER

Neck Exercises

In a comfortable position, either standing or sitting, take a deep breath. Without moving the shoulders, roll the head slowly and directly backward toward the spine. Now, very slowly, exhale and bring the head forward until the chin rests as close as possible to the chest. Repeat this movement several times, always moving the head as slowly as possible, and always deep breathing.

With the head in an upright position, inhale and slowly turn the head to the right as far as it is comfortably possible. Exhale and return the head to the front and center.

Now inhale and slowly turn the head to the left side. Exhale and return the head to the front and center. Remember to refrain from any shoulder movement, and police yourself constantly to keep from going too fast. Repeat the exercises several times.

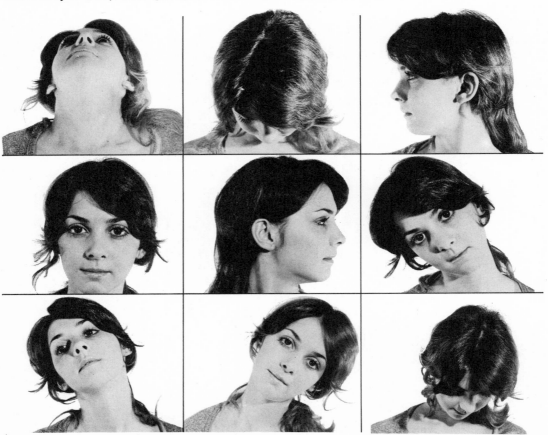

YOGA REWARDS THOSE WHO PERSEVERE

Tilt the head to the right side as though seeking to touch the ear to the shoulder, and inhale. Do not move the body; only the neck and head are in movement. Exhale and return the head to the front position. Repeat several times, and relax.

Perform this same movement, including the deep breathing, toward the left side and then relax.

Now taking a deep breath, slowly rotate the neck to the right as though it were on well greased ball-bearings. Deep breathe in and out very slowly. Keep the shoulders straight and move only the head and neck. Very slowly allow the head to swivel from the front center position all the way around until it is returned to the front center. Relax.

Now repeat this exercise by rotating the head to the left.

Waking Up Exercise

Yoga teaches us never to shock the body. And yet in the course of a day we apply innumerable shocks to our nervous system.

One of our greatest offenses to our body is committed as soon as we open our eyes, in the way we arouse ourselves. Usually we choose to remain in bed until the last possible moment before we suddenly panic and realize it is growing late. We jump from the bed at that moment and apply the first shock of the day to our body. As our feet thud to the floor, we jar our entire nervous system. In this manner, we set the tone for the remaining hours of the day.

From this shattering awakening, tension will build and climb, for the body has been thrust rather brutally into action instead of being permitted to gain momentum gradually. This in turn negates the night's rest that would have served its purpose of helping the body to begin the day in a relaxed condition.

Compare our usual awakening to that of an animal. The animal slowly stretches its entire body, yawns, and is up and ready for activity immediately following that.

Next, observe a baby as it awakens. It follows the same sensible pattern as the animal. Even if his awakening comes from hunger pains, first the baby stretches his arms and legs. Only after that will he respond to the sharp hunger pains and begin to shriek. Even stronger, then, than the hunger pains is nature's natural way of awakening.

We also used to awaken in this manner. But as we became sophisticated and rushed, we lost or gave up this delightful awakening of the body.

The following technique of awakening gradually is the only Yoga exercise that we shall perform in bed. But by taking a few moments to perform this movement, a beneficial change will begin to take place in the body. There will be an improvement to the disposition; a cheerfulness and alertness that will be considered unusual in some will gradually come about.

By avoiding the usual shock into which we thrust our bodies upon awakening, the body in turn will respond by sidestepping that first tension-builder of the day and performing more serenely.

To practice the Waking Up exercise, lie on your back with your arms comfortably by your sides. Take a deep breath and raise the right leg a few inches from the bed and stretch it to its fullest length. Exhale as you lower your leg. Relax.

Now raise the left leg and repeat the movement, deep breathing just as with the right leg. Relax a moment and raise both legs and stretch them, deep breathing in and out. Relax.

Inhale and raise both arms behind the head and stretch them. Exhale and relax. Now inhale and raise both the arms and the legs only a few inches above the mattress level and stretch in both directions. While your arms and legs are suspended, rotate the wrists and ankles in a clockwise, and then counter-clockwise movement. Exhale and relax.

This entire exercise takes only a couple of minutes. And yet the tenor of your whole day may be dependent on it.

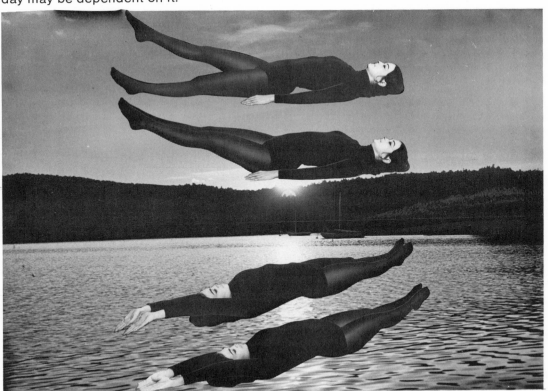

YOGA REWARDS THOSE WHO PERSEVERE

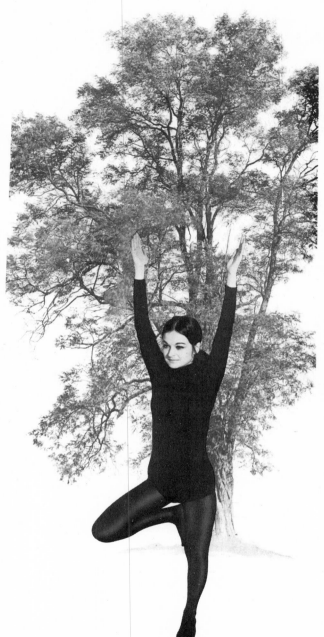

The Tree

As with many other Yoga asanas, the Tree posture takes its name from its resemblance to some inert or active part of nature. In the first step of the Tree, find a comfortable standing position. Concentrate on a spot on the wall in front of you. THis will help to create your equilibrium, or balance of body, as you attempt the pose.

Keeping the left leg straight and unbending, bring the foot of the right leg to rest on the upper, inner thigh of the left leg as you deep breathe very slowly in and out. Try to place the right foot as close to the crotch as possible.

Arms should be raised overhead and pointing skyward. Hold this position for two or three minutes if possible. Then change positions and try the same posture standing on the right foot.

Because of stiffness or oversize thighs, many people cannot bring their feet to rest against the upper thigh in the beginning. When this is the case, place the foot on the calf or on the knee at the most comfortable spot. With continued daily practice, you will be able to place the foot higher and higher until eventually the knee will bend agilely and the foot will easily reach the upper thigh.

EXERCISES AND BENEFITS IN CHAPTER 3

Head to Knee—This reaching posture stimulates the entire body in addition to limbering the spine. The upper arms receive toning along with the abdomen. In addition, all posterior muscles are flexed and bulges are removed. An excellent movement for easing indigestion discomfort.

Squatting—The benefits of squatting are an aid to good posture and a limbering of the knees. Balance is improved by the slow descent to the position of sitting on the heels.

Neck Exercises—These varied and soothing movements offer many and lasting benefits. The tension of the body that settles in the neck area is diminished in proportion to the application of these exercises.
There is usually an improvement in vision after practicing these exercises for a period of time. Increased blood circulation to the ophthalmic nerves brings this about.

Waking Up Exercises—The perfect way to commence a day. By avoiding the shock of jumping from bed into immediate activity, the body gradually adjusts to movement after hours of rest. A must for daily arising.

The Tree—The first step of the Tree leads into a posture practiced for its balancing benefits. Mastery of this simple asana will combat a tendency toward motion sickness and a fear of high places. This discipline is achieved by teaching oneself the method of maintaining perfect self-balance.

YOGA REWARDS THOSE WHO PERSEVERE

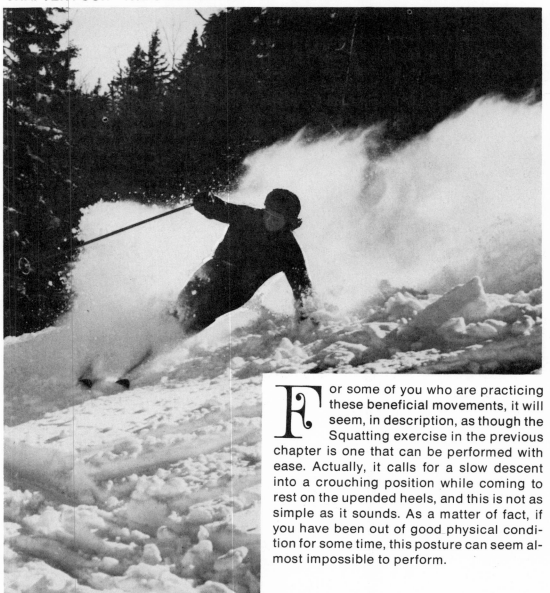

For some of you who are practicing these beneficial movements, it will seem, in description, as though the Squatting exercise in the previous chapter is one that can be performed with ease. Actually, it calls for a slow descent into a crouching position while coming to rest on the upended heels, and this is not as simple as it sounds. As a matter of fact, if you have been out of good physical condition for some time, this posture can seem almost impossible to perform.

And yet, in the course of daily living, we very much need to use this convenient posture. The fact that we have moved our body in positions related to this, and yet find the Squatting position difficult, shows us that we need more than the usual routine of work to bring our bodies back to good shape and use.

In this position, we can check through various drawers in file cabinets or place things in storage space under a kitchen counter, squat to play with a child, and tend to our garden with greater agility. Or if we choose to be contemplative, we can study the industry of an ant at close range.

Why should the delight of folding our bodies into a compact, serviceable unit be lost to us? It is really a sensible, satisfying posture to hold, bringing grace and balance to an uncertain body.

In the islands of the Caribbean and the Mediterranean, the natives can sit at work all day in the squatting position. In the open market stalls, one sees serene and comfortable people squatting by the hour, never tiring, and never uncomfortable. They have stretched their leg muscles to a rewarding degree that permits them an extended use of their body.

Of course, they began to use this position when they were young, for in the islands and in the Far Eastern countries, the debilitating Western comfort found in the soft chairs we use is fortunately still comparatively unknown. When these agile people rise and walk, it is with assurance and poise, for their bodies perform for, instead of against, them.

Without doubt, this squatting exercise can be very demanding for our Western society. Although you may not choose to spend your leisure or business time in this position, you will notice increased agility returning to your hip area after repeated practice of Squatting II.

Helen was a natural and self taught skier. Growing up in the snowy New England states, she had skied with the same abandon and skill as an islander riding the surf. But this had all been years ago, before Helen's family had put new demands on her attention and time.

In addition, Helen no longer had an impressive slope just outside her door. In consequence of her duties and the distance to the nearest slopes, Helen daydreamed of skiing, but could not fit the activity into her plans.

Special arrangements were made for a birthday treat for Helen that included a weekend of skiing in the mountains. She was dismayed to find that she no longer could sweep through the powdery snow with the abandon of her earlier years. The whole weekend was a disappointment and an ordeal.

"I seemed to have lost my confidence in my own body, though I spent years on skis," Helen lamented. "Coming down those slopes that weekend, I knew I had lost something that was important to me; a sense of ease with my movements, and an ability to command my body. Even though I thought I was in good shape from swimming, tennis, and general calisthenics, my early control of my body movements was gone."

Helen began to practice Yoga. She faithfully allowed a minimum of fifteen minutes a day for the exercises. By the time the first snows had covered the nearby Poconos Mountains, Helen was en route up the trail. She returned from her weekend glowing with pleasure.

"It was the Squatting on flat feet that did it," she said. "Though all the asanas helped me regain control over my body, the Squatting put me back on skis."

Actually, the benefits of the Squatting exercises aren't limited to skiers by any means. When this position is taken daily and repeated slowly two or three times, difficulties of elimination can be corrected. It is also an aid in preventing constipation.

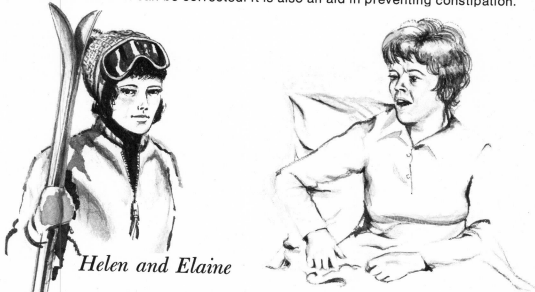

Helen and Elaine

Elaine was a chronic complainer. "My back hurts today," she would announce. Or perhaps it was, "I have a stiff neck." At times it was a generalized complaint her friends and family heard: "I don't feel so well today."

Though most everyone sympathized with Elaine, she really was not very pleasant company. When she visited someone, she always asked for a cushion to wedge behind her back and a footstool on which to rest her aching feet. Or she would go around the room testing the various chairs, moving from one to another as discomfort commenced. Hostesses developed a feeling of guilt because they could not provide comfort for Elaine. She was not a popular guest.

Doctors found nothing seriously wrong with Elaine's back, and referred to her discomfort simply as a weak back. Finally, one of the many doctors she consulted suggested that she might benefit from some form of exercise that strengthened the back muscles.

Elaine began doing mild calisthenics which seemed to benefit her condition. She continued the exercises for some time before deciding that she was not an athletic or even an active type of person, and that this had led to her weakness in the first place. She knew she had to have some form of regular exercise, so she turned to Yoga because of its moderate and understated movements.

Six weeks after Elaine began practicing the Rock and Roll, Waking Up, and the Cobra, among others, she found she could get through an entire day without the dull protest from her back that she had experienced for so many years.

What seemed to do the most for her?

"The Cobra. When I first tried to roll my head and take my spine into a backward curl, I couldn't even get my entire neck off the floor. I was almost paralyzed stiff, and that was the condition of my spine. I didn't force it, though. Day after day I went through the same movements, and didn't seem to move my spine an inch. But eventually it came."

Slow, determined and intelligent restraint had its rewards. Elaine, through easy but frequent movement, returned her spinal column and its surrounding muscles and ligaments to good working condition. It was a steady improvement, and because the posture was carefully achieved, Elaine never tired from the position.

Janie was an attractive woman for whom one automatically felt a sense of pity. Her beautiful face and delicate hands and feet seemed to emphasize her abnormally heavy stomach. In the beginning of her classes, Janie even wore a rigid girdle under her bulging leotards. Sensitive to her bulk in this area, Janie had tried to conceal as much of it as possible under an old-fashioned and tortuously laced up contraption.

Janie's husband, taking the course in Yoga with her, was slender and flat stomached. And yet Janie always appeared to be trying to hide behind or to the side of him.

Persuaded she could not possibly move her body to its benefit under such restrictions as the girdle, Janie came to the next class corsetless and red of face. But she was determined to rescue her body. Both she and her husband never missed a class. Week after week they came and while Don swept easily through his exercises, Janie struggled to roll, tried to reach her toes, attempted to stand on one leg with the other

THE SKIER'S EXERCISE THAT'S GOOD FOR EVERYONE

tucked against her thigh, and finally, tried to reach her ankles behind her as she went into the Bow posture.

But the protruding stomach always seemed to get in the way. Her knees could not come near her chest in the Rock and Roll. The heavy bulge prevented her from reaching beyond her knees, a long distance from the desired goal of the toes. Over and over she tried to bring her legs over her buttocks as she attempted to do the Bow. But it was as though she were teetering on a ball—a constant struggle.

But Janie was valiant, and she had a goal. Not once did she complain, and there was not one exercise that she did not attempt. Her husband remained attentive to her plight and helped her with frequent expressions of encouragement. And he grew more lithe, and stood straighter, and seemed to be enjoying a sense of well-being.

Lectures on nutrition were included in the Yoga class. Janie listened and took notes and began to bring in original recipes she had tried from the various whole grains, nuts, and fresh fruits and vegetables which she was now including in their diet.

She continued to struggle with the exercises. And her persistence eventually paid off. The abdomen began to shrink. By the end of the course, she had regained a greater use of her body. But she repeated the course as a beginner when the first ten weeks were over. This time she was alone.

"I need the discipline," she said.

Janie

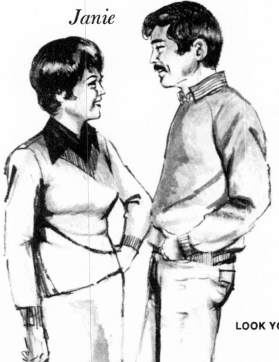

Janie arrived each week with a conspiratorial eager-to-share expression.

"Another inch this week off my waistline."

"Down another inch and a half."

"My skirts are falling off of me."

And Janie's abdomen continued to disappear. It was not a swift action. Even after five months, Janie still had work to do. But she had come so far that now she was within sight of her goal of a beautiful and functional body.

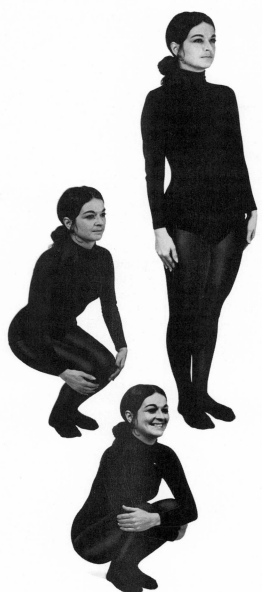

Squatting With the Feet Flat On the Floor

In a standing position, with the arms by the side, take a deep breath. Exhale as you slowly lower your body to a squatting position. Keep the feet flat on the floor and resist a tendency to bring the heels upward.

The upper torso will slant forward in this movement in order to achieve the proper balance. The thighs will press against the abdomen as you assume the correct posture. Your arms may be held loosely before you, with the elbow area coming to rest upon the knees as you reach the ultimate position.

Breathe in and out, and try to hold this stance for a minute or two. In the beginning, it will probably not be a very comfortable position in which to remain. But as your legs stretch and as the knees become more flexible, you will begin to understand why certain people around the world instinctively fall into this position when wanting to rest, but not wanting to recline.

This is a splendid movement for skiers, as it strengthens the ankles and thigh muscles. If exercise of this area has been neglected during the year, it is a good idea for those who will be heading for the ski slopes to commence practicing Squatting I and II in the fall months in order to gain the agility and balance required for remaining upright on skis when doing the slalom.

The Cobra in its back-bending movements gently flexes and massages each vertebra of the spine. Included in this motion is a complete stretching of the neck, shoulders, spine, and buttocks. Tone is

THE SKIER'S EXERCISE THAT'S GOOD FOR EVERYONE

given to the lower back muscles, and as the head and shoulders lift up and roll backward, the entire abdominal area is flattened in movement, bringing tone to this part of the body, too.

That area between the abdomen and the chest, commonly called the breadbasket, and often resembling just that, receives a very helpful tautening.

Actually, in posture, the Cobra does resemble the reptile for which it is named. The rolling backward of the head should be accomplished with the same ease that a cobra would use in its own movement, and when you perform it, allow no sudden rearing back of the shoulders.

There should be no rush to perfect this posture. First of all, for many it may be an unaccustomed movement of the body. Secondly, a gradual return to the spinal litheness is more desirable than an attempt to overcome spinal rigidity too rapidly. Yoga, performed correctly, is never a sudden movement, nor an extreme one. It is a leading of the body into its maximum efficiency at a reasonable rate of speed.

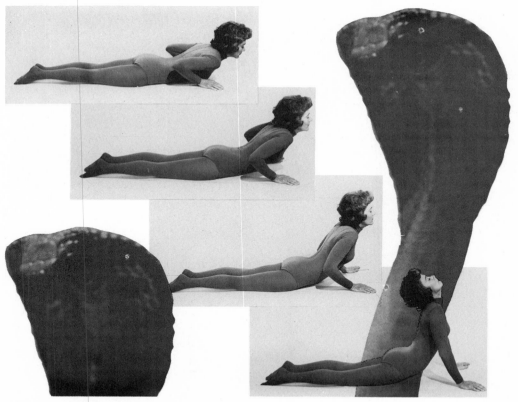

Cobra I

Lie face down in a prone position on the floor, with the palms spread flat on the floor just below shoulder level. Take a deep breath and bring the head and back up very slowly. The flatly spread hands—still on the floor—will help to support the body as it rolls slowly backward. Perform this movement with restraint, without any sudden or forceful action.

Hold this backward body bend for a moment before exhaling and slowly lowering the body until it rests flat once again.

Another version of the Cobra can be performed following the Cobra I. In Cobra II, take the same position as in Cobra I. Take a deep breath and bring the head and back up very slowly, without support of the hands. The hands will rise at the same time that the face is lifted, and they will turn palms frontward, the same as the face. Continue to roll the head and shoulders backward as far as is comfortable, exhale and come down.

An important concept in Yoga is learning to control body movements. We are accustomed to brevity in our actions. We lie down, sit down, stand, or walk, and limit ourselves, generally, to moving within this circumscribed framework. With such restricted motion of the body, there are bound to be areas that are not flexed or exercised, and in consequence, grow stiffened from lack of use.

The Boat offers a discipline coming from concentration, among its other attributes. There is constant defiance from the body when this posture is taken. The folded arms tend to cup the head, and the legs fight their unsupported pose, But daily practice of the Boat eventually brings about healthy discipline and at the same time supplies the physical needs of the body.

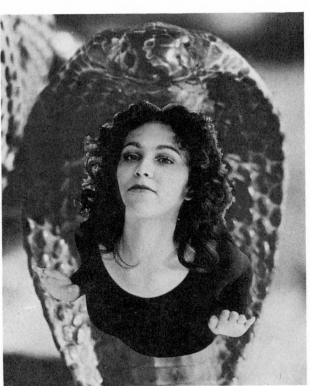

THE SKIER'S EXERCISE THAT'S GOOD FOR EVERYONE

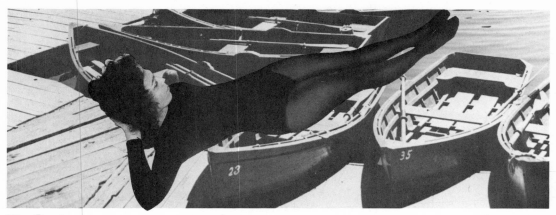

The Boat

Lie flat on the floor on your back. Interlock the fingers behind the head, just above the neck in a supportive fashion. Keep the elbows straight and do not permit them to cup the head. Taking a deep breath, raise the head, shoulders, and legs upward from the floor to a height not exceeding a foot. Keep the knees straight. Hold this position for a moment before exhaling and returning to a prone position on the floor.

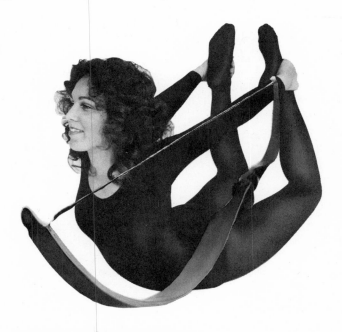

The Bow

Putting to use the very practical science of Hatha Yoga, when the body is bent in one direction, there is an opposite stretch to balance the scales. The Bow offers an excellent means of creating a beneficial bending of the back, after the curving of the spine in the Boat. With many Yogic postures, the name of the pose suggests the animal, bird, or action for which it is named. The asana is aptly called, for it does indeed resemble an archer's bow.

Lie on the stomach flat on the floor. Bend the knees and bring the legs over the back. Reach backward with the hands and take hold of the ankles. Try for a firm grasp. Take a deep breath and raise the head and the knees as far above the floor as you can. Exhale and come down.

In the beginning, it may not be possible to lift the knees off the floor to create the curve of a bow. Don't despair. After all, it has probably been many years since these specific muscles, tendons, and ligaments have been called into play. Go at this slowly, not looking for day to day advances in movements, but rather, continue a steady daily exercising schedule that will eventually bring the results that you want.

EXERCISE BENEFITS IN CHAPTER 4

Squatting II—With the Feet Flat On the Floor called the skier's exercise, this second squatting position strengthens the ankles and thigh muscles. Great emphasis is placed also on the excellent benefits in helping to prevent constipation. The asana is noted further as an excellent posture for elimination.

Cobra—The back bending position is used for relieving tension and backache. Muscles and ligaments near the spine are treated to an easy massage in this exercise that aims at rolling the head backward along the spine for several inches.
An added merit to the Cobra posture is its tautening effect on sagging buttocks. But go at this exercise slowly and cautiously, never straining for an impressive position. Rather, rise easily and naturally, allowing the back to gain its elasticity through practice instead of force.
If there is any tendency toward complete rigidity on the spine, this posture must be approached with caution. Once commenced, in such cases, the exercise should require a longer period of time to perfect.

The Boat—The abdominal muscles are strengthened and abdominal fat is reduced by this posture. The Boat also relieves constipation. The shoulders, back, and pelvic region are brought into play and toned.

The Bow—Benefits of the Bow are many. Because of its curved position, this posture affects the glands beneficially. It is sometimes referred to as "The Internal Massage." Since the posture involves lying on the stomach, grasping the feet behind the back and gently drawing them in toward the head in a bow shape, it arches and strengthens the chest and abdominal area. The Bow is used also to relieve a tendency toward flatulence.

CHAPTER FIVE - AN ASANA FOR WHATEVER'S AILING YOU

he dedicated practice of Yoga never fails to bring a grab-bag of surprises to the practitioner. And it is always with gratification and reconfirmed faith that a teacher hears a student speak in wonder of the physical and mental changes taking place in his body as he progresses in the practice of Hatha Yoga.

The instructor knows that within days, or weeks at the most, a formerly distressed student will begin to rise above the effects of sedentary living. But the newcomer to Yoga speaks of the welcome changes happening to him as though a near miracle were occurring, which it could well be considered.

This is especially true when the person enjoying the new expansion of his physical abilities is an aged arthritic; or even a young person afflicted with this disease. One hears the almost unbelieving, "I can open and close my hands for the first time in years." Or "I have gone back up to my bedroom to sleep, now that my knees permit me to climb a flight of stairs again." Another familiar phrase is "I've grown so peaceful these days. I can actually look at every member of my family without wanting to lash out at anyone."

These assertions are all testimonials to the effectiveness of Yoga as a tool for both physical and mental rehabilitation. Usually the good effects felt by someone practicing this discipline for the first time open up a whole new plane of existence, restoring him to a more useful level of function as a human being.

With these carefully worked-out exercises, one can rid himself of long-standing discomforts or mental depression that condemns him to an unexciting and tiresome existence. It is by taking part in these exercises, by applying the simple Yoga discipline to one's own life, that a casual course-taker becomes a serious enthusiast for healthful and active living.

The lessons in this chapter bring about the near miracles which have changed the health and lives of so many persons. With steady day-to-day practice of the beginning exercises, Yoga becomes an upward reaching ladder that offers itself as a means of attaining the degree of activity and the peak of health and beauty that is each person's right.

Because each individual must decide the rate at which he advances from one lesson to another, there is no regular plan of performance. One should attempt to practice all the postures, and to continue interest in them even as one moves on to others. The exercises may be spread out over as long a period of time as one desires.

Instead of learning to live with one's malfunctioning body, there should be a tremendous desire to overcome any and all afflictions that assault it. Abject acceptance of one's ills begins the sure and steady decline into the destructive processes of aging. To permit the body to submit to afflictions brought on by under- or over-active glands or organs is senseless, and a crime committed on the body.

Yoga provides the means for alleviating even major discomforts, and restoring the body to better health. Given a chance, hardly anyone will fail to respond to the gentle massaging movements of Yoga. In fact, even a wheelchair patient can respond to the benefits of some mild Hatha Yoga movements. The hands can be used to increase circulation in this area and the impressive neck and shoulder exercises will restore agility to stiffened muscles. There is always some asana that can help nearly anyone. Neither age nor limited physical mobility should deter you from taking the rewarding path of healthful exercise.

Fay was a handsome woman in her fifties when she first decided she would submit to the entreaties of her friends and begin to practice the Yoga discipline. With an underactive thyroid which required daily medication to enable her to combat a serious weight problem, Fay had decided there was nothing that could free her from a life-long program of pill taking. For 20 years she had accepted this adjunct to her day, with gratitude for the effectiveness of the medicine, but with a natural resentment toward the condition which controlled her body.

Fay was exhausted much of the time, and there were days when she chose not to get out of bed.

"I was tired, and the effort to move about seemed too great. Why should I get up? I'd merely find a chair somewhere and proceed to sit there for hours, growing more fatigued than if I remained in bed."

It was a slow path of improvement for Fay when she began to practice her Rock and Rolls. She was determined to give every opportunity to these body movements to see if they would indeed do for her what her friends said.

In the beginning, she almost gave up in despair. Her friends advanced with enthusiasm from one exercise to the next, seeming to come more alive with each week's practice. But Fay felt little if any change for the better.

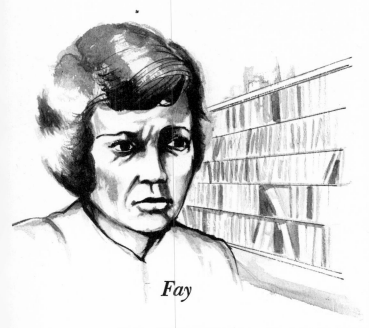

Fay

She had tried so very many things to help remove this physical exhaustion, but nothing so far had helped.

Her library was full of books on self-helps that so far had not removed the fatigue with which she awakened nearly every morning, and which followed her throughout the day.

Fay had begun to develop an indifferent attitude about her condition that was affecting her attitude toward life in general. Because she was an intelligent woman and one with a wide range of interests, she had not wanted to accept this condition passively.

So without too much hope, but because she was determined to give this discipline every chance, Fay persisted and went from one set of exercises to another. And then one day she began to practice the shoulder stand. That day and the next and the next, there was some sense of elevation to her spirits as she lay resting between exercises.

Encouraged, Fay applied herself enthusiastically to her daily asanas. Now she was advancing into more demanding postures. But it was always the shoulder stand to which she looked forward.

"It was as though I'd just had a satisfying meal, or had been invigorated, as one might be from taking a walk after several hours of sitting still."

In the mornings, as soon as Fay awakened, she learned to lie on the floor beside the bed and go into a shoulder stand. She did no other exercise in the early morning hours, for she found her body too protesting. But there was a strong compulsion to practice the shoulder stand every morning.

Toward the end of her course Fay was radiant with news one day.

"I went to the doctor's for my physical check-up this week, and he discharged me! He said I had apparently reactivated my thyroid by practicing the shoulder stand. He says my condition should remain improved as long as I practice the shoulder stand for several minutes each day."

Fay's position in the shoulder stand had directed a fresh and invigorated blood supply toward her sluggish thyroid gland. This stimulating action allowed the gland to resume its duties of controlling the metabolism and standing guard over the physical and mental processes of the body.

Lisa was a young woman with an old posture. All her life she recalled feeling more comfortable in a slouch than standing in an upright position. There was something defensive in her posture as she curled her shoulders around the sides of her chest and created a near hollow in this region.

What might have been an attractive young person was distorted into a round-shouldered woman whose appearance was one of age and exhaustion. For in this position, it is impossible to breathe correctly, and in consequence, Lisa's complexion was a splotchy brown, further emphasizing the look of despair that she wore constantly.

"My mother is always ordering me to stand up straight, and telling me my complexion resembles a mud-hen. So I straighten my shoulders for a few minutes, but before I know it, they're slumped down again."

Lisa had no place else to go, and nothing to do with her evenings. But because she had not completely accepted her lonely state and unattractive appearance, she was looking for some means of aiding her distressed body.

Lisa showed improvement almost from the beginning once she began practicing Yoga movements. Though she didn't straighten her shoulders overnight, she did begin to work consciously at her basic problem of posture. Deep breathing was an excellent reminder to hold her shoulders upright. And because this was an unobtrusive exercise that could be practiced at any time of the day without calling attention to itself, Lisa was able to perform deep-breathing exercises at her desk off and on throughout the day.

But it was when she found the Dolphin and realized it fitted her needs that Lisa was able to concentrate on correcting her problem of rounded shoulders. The exercise was an uncomfortable one for her, with her particular problem. Each time she relaxed after doing this asana, she would have to massage her shoulders, because muscles and ligaments that had not been much used were being called into play again. Tone was beginning to develop in the shoulder area and the upper arms and neck were receiving their benefits from this stretching movement.

In time, with daily practicing of the Dolphin and the other asanas, Lisa developed an attractive carriage and lost her cowed posture. Her skin, too, shed its muddy tones, as once again it was bathed from within by a strong blood supply, brought about by a good oxygen intake, now that the breathing organ was put to full use.

While all Yoga exercises are good to practice, and offer a multitude of benefits, sometimes it seems as though a specific Yoga movement works like a prescription for an individual. Just as the shoulder stand brought a more perfectly working thyroid to Fay, and the Dolphin helped to correct Lisa's posture and complexion problems, so the Plough seemed to be the answer to Frances' difficulties.

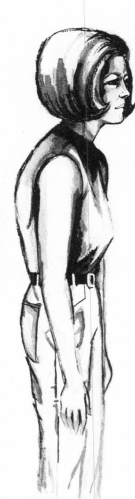

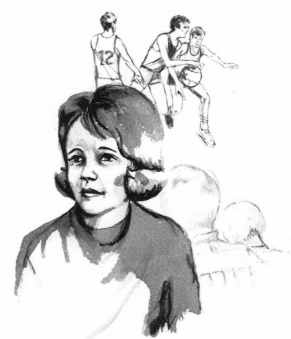

Lisa and Frances

Frances was yet another woman who had grown old before her time. One was not positive she had ever really been young, in the sense of having a supple spine, an ease of movement in bending, sitting, or rising from a chair.

Frances had never liked sports activities, and took no part in voluntary exercise. During her school days, she came to class with written excuses as to why she should not take part in gym activities. The family doctor had been pressured into saying Frances was not capable of participating in any form of calisthenics.

In those earlier years, Frances had been young. But she had also been lazy. It was most likely a diet lacking in nutrition that sent her to school wanting to conserve all her scant energy. Or perhaps it was just a bad habit into which she had fallen. But Frances, in her late twenties, had the movements of a fragile, older woman whose agility had disappeared with her youth.

Though Frances was young in years, she was stiff of back and discouraged with her own lack of enthusiasm for living. Had she followed her original path of neglect for the moving parts of her body, Frances would surely have been headed for an early debilitating malady, since stiffened joints develop from such indifference. And more than one nursing home has as its occupant a young, wheelchair patient who began to ruin her body early in life through complete neglect.

Frances had seen such cases herself when she went to visit an older relative in a nursing home. And it was after such a visit that she realized this was the route she was travelling.

In Yoga, one improvement in the body usually leads to another. For example, when one learns to deep-breathe correctly and take in sufficient oxygen, the blood supply is hastened in its movements. This stimulates a sluggish bloodstream and helps to bring renewed life through oxygen nourishment.

Once stimulated, a body can move more easily. This creates a desire for more action, which brings, in its own turn, a need for more nutrition. This is why Yoga teaches that for the best results, the study, practice and understanding of good nutrition must be incorporated into the practice of Yoga.

As Frances practiced her physical movements for a minimum of fifteen minutes a day, she never failed to accompany them with deep breathing. The life stream of blood was carried less reluctantly to all parts of her body as her increased physical activity pumped it through. And life in Frances began to stir.

It was the performance of the Plough that brought Frances the greatest pleasure. Daily practice of this asana gave her the suppleness she had lost early in life. As she rolled her spine backward until her toes touched the floor behind her head, she never ceased to exult in her own prowess and in her now agile spine. And then, with the physical Yoga, Frances was introduced to Yoga's beliefs about eating only natural foods.

Her counter breakfasts of orange juice, toast and coffee were replaced with whole grain cereals and honey, or protein-rich eggs and fruit. Her sandwich lunches were given up and she began to take thermos bottles of rich vegetable soups to work with fruit and nuts for added energy. In the evenings she took the time to prepare simple but nourishing meals. She became a young woman restored to good health through a sensible plan of exercise and good eating.

Shoulder Stand

Lie comfortably flat on the back with the arms by the side, and take a deep breath. Raise both legs together while keeping the knees straight. Check them as they rise to avoid a natural tendency to bend.

After achieving a 90° angle with the legs, place the hands under the hips. Continue the upward movement, and with the help of the hands, raise the torso in the air so that

AN ASANA FOR WHATEVER'S AILING YOU

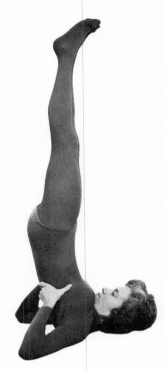

only the shoulders and head remain in contact with the floor.

The spine must be kept straight. The chin will press against the chest after the legs are in the air and the spine is erect. As the hips rise into the air, the hands must support the upper back rather than the hips or even the waist. There is a tendency, in the beginning, to allow the hands to remain in supporting position at the waist. Check this position frequently as you first practice the Shoulder Stand. If the hands do not press toward the upper back, above the waist, then the spine does not receive sufficient support, and in consequence, the posture is not correct.

Keep the legs relaxed and avoid any tenseness.

Lower the legs slowly by "walking" the hands down the sides of the spine until your body is flat on the floor again. Do not drop your legs suddenly from this upright position.

For those experiencing difficulty in performing the Shoulder Stand, learn to roll the body backward as you lie on the floor. Keeping the shoulders flat, attempt to roll the legs and torso backward until you can raise the legs above your body, remembering to support the spine at all times with the hands placed above the waist. Correct placement of the hands is vital in retaining a straight back position.

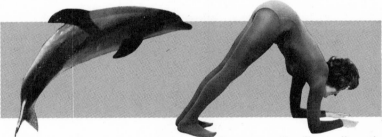

The Dolphin

Take a position on the hands and knees. Then place the elbows on the floor directly in front of the knees. Now take a small knee-step backward. Deep breathe as you go up on your toes, and straighten your knees. The hands and elbows remain flat on the floor. Do not allow the elbows to leave their contact with the floor. The weight of the body must be on the arms and toes. Lift the head upward as high as possible. Exhale and return knees to the floor.

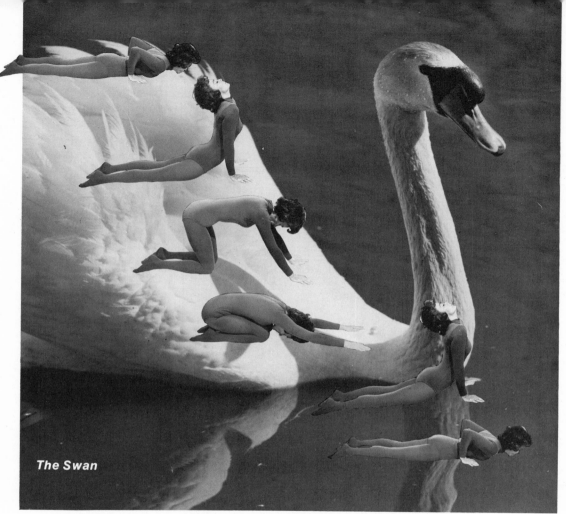

The Swan

Lie on the abdomen in a completely straight position. Place the palms flat on the floor and close to the waist. Deep breathe and raise the head, shoulders, chest and abdomen; until the weight of this part of the body is on the arms. The legs remain on the floor. Poise the head up and back as far as possible. Exhale and bring the buttocks backward, bending at both the hips and the knees, until the abdomen is pressing flat against the thighs, and the buttocks are on the heels. The head is now dropped downward and the hands do not move.

Inhale and bring the body forward until the weight is once again on the arms and legs. Exhale and drop the body to a prone position on the floor.

AN ASANA FOR WHATEVER'S AILING YOU

The Plough

Lie flat on the floor, on the back, with both arms lying by the sides. In a backward roll, bring both legs upward while keeping the knees perfectly straight. Do not permit them to bend.

Take a deep breath, and holding the knees completely straight, bring them to a point just above the face. Roll on backward until the toes touch the floor in back of the head.

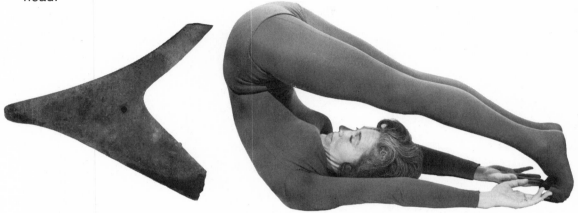

Exhale and return the legs to the original prone position on the floor, remembering to keep the knees straight at all times.

In all of these Yoga positions, it is good discipline to remain in position as long as is comfortably possible. Of course, you should release your body from any movement or position before bringing discomfort. But one of the ideals of Yoga is to work toward non-movement of the body, or the ability to control and maintain comfort in any beneficial position.

EXERCISE BENEFITS IN CHAPTER 5

Shoulder Stand—This is one of the most important of all Yogic postures in its effect on blood circulation. The increased blood supply creates a beautifying effect on the skin, and continued practice of this posture stimulates the secretions of the sex glands which create a youthful appearance.

The Shoulder Stand is especially helpful in stimulating the natural function of the thyroid gland. Proper weight control can be managed in this way, and any body action controlled by the thyroid can be speeded up.

The Dolphin—This is an excellent shoulder and arm strengthener. It is also helpful in preparing for the Head Stand. More immediate results will be found in the correction of poor posture. The upward movement of the head, taken while the arms and legs support the body in its slanted lift, brings a fresh blood supply to the face for an increase in both health and beauty. An ideal posture for removing tension.

The upper arms and shoulders receive toning from this position, and in addition, there is a pull on lazy shoulders that slope or curve. The chest area also is stretched and allowed to develop a more normal breathing pattern.

The Swan—The Swan teaches fluidity of movement as it takes the crouched body backward in a slow glide to rest briefly in a prone position before returning to its original arched stance. In this exercise any tendency toward rounded shoulders and hollow chest is corrected as the straightening and flattening pull on the upper torso is gently exerted. The accordion-like movement of the body is greatly beneficial to the peristaltic action of the intestines, and therefore aids in preventing constipation.

The Swan has been found by many to be sleep-conducive if practiced slowly a few times before retiring. Or if sleep is long in coming and is accompanied by a sense of restlessness, it has been found helpful to leave the bed and practice this movement several times before returning to bed. It would seem that the gentle flexing and stretching, accompanied as it is by the soothing fetal position, prepares the body for natural, easy sleep.

The Plough—The Plough, in appearance, resembles the ancient piece of Indian equipment for which it was named. Complete flexibility of the spine is achieved by this movement. Those with a tendency toward arthritis will find relief in the increased elasticity of the spine brought about by the limbering movement. In addition, the thyroid gland is stimulated by the angled posture. This position can even measure your degree of youth, as related to a supple spine.

If the completed position can be achieved without strain, then the entire vertebral column is in excellent condition. For those experiencing difficulty achieving this position, slow and gentle exercises for the spine, such as the Rock and Roll movement, are indicated to help restore the natural elasticity. Added benefits of the Plough include a beautifying effect on the complexion which comes from overall body stimulation.

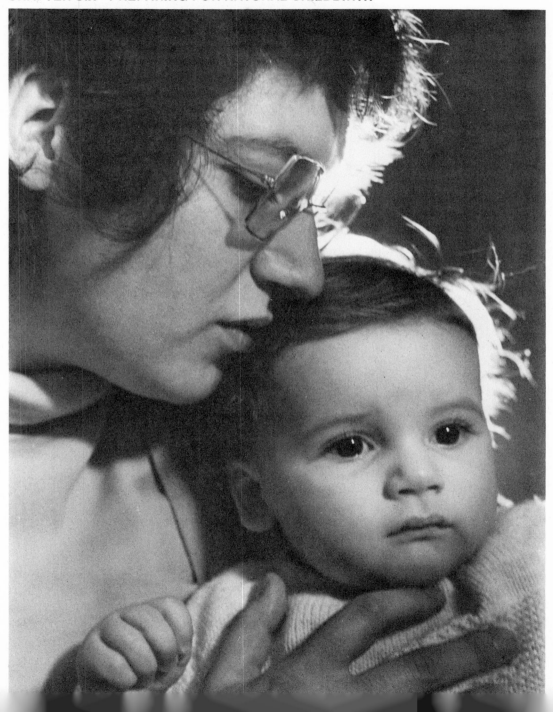

Natural childbirth is becoming more common because of its growing appeal to young women who are convinced that an undrugged birth gives more advantages to both child and mother. There is a quicker recovery for the mother, and a less traumatic experience for the infant, in this method of delivery than in those births employing sedatives and anesthesia.

Without anesthesia, delivery is swifter, less complicated, and—according to those who experience it—brings far more satisfaction to the mother who actually remains awake and assists in her own delivery. Discomfort and pain are minimized, if during the months preceding the birth, the mother engages in some form of planned exercise combined with deep breathing.

Because of the established benefits of this drugless delivery, young women interested in giving every possible chance to their unborn child are looking for means to prepare for the event.

Some doctors have approved the practice of Hatha Yoga as a means of adding tone to those areas of the body that will be called upon to work the hardest in childbirth. If all parts of the body are getting sufficient and complete exercise on a daily basis, rather than a sporadic basis, natural childbirth can be a rewarding and inspiring event.

Thorough preparation for such a delivery is essential. When expectant mothers enter a Yoga class, their efforts should be directed mainly toward developing and strengthening the pelvic area. Any leg movement is desirable for bringing tone to the expectant mother's body. For upon her physical condition and suppleness will depend the ease of the experience before her.

No one wants to suffer. And knowing that a flexible body will determine their future degree of comfort, these women should undertake their preparation with serious intent.

One obstetrician, when asked about the wisest preparation for childbirth, had surprising things to say. He suggested that the woman who fares the best during this experience is the one who might not have been overjoyed at the prospect of having a child, and consequently, works toward concealing the fact that she is pregnant for as long as possible.

This would mean, he said, that she holds her stomach in at all times without permitting a slouch to develop which would push her abdomen out. She exercises with dedication to prevent excess weight and poor muscle tone from pulling her body further out of shape. In addition, she watches her diet and eliminates all foods of a non-essential nature.

According to the obstetrician, this type of mother delivers with a minimum of discomfort, for she has not been carrying a child unnecessarily large, as she would if she ate without restriction. She therefore has an easy delivery. Her own recovery, moreover, is rapid because her body is not burdened with the usual weight gain so familiar to new mothers.

The woman who fares less well is the one who takes such pride in her enceinte condition that she commences wearing maternity frocks almost immediately, whether she requires them or not. This is conducive, according to the doctor, to easy expansion of the stomach in a sense of pride. With the smock or blouselike dress concealing the appearance of the abdominal area, there is less inclination to stand erect and provide the support—that this part of the body will grow increasingly to need—by using the spine as a regulator of posture.

Not only will this attitude create a more difficult delivery, but after the birth of the child, the condition that was created during the preceding months will exact its toll in back pain and other distresses. The mother must remember that the event of childbirth will not end with the birth of her child. She will be picking up her baby and tending it in the months following its birth. Therefore, she must ensure the fact that she has developed a strong back, and a body that will allow her to care for her child with ease.

Women who choose natural delivery without the aid of injections to dull them to the sensation of giving birth, or to render them unconscious at this great moment, invariably have subsequent children by the same method; a proof of its practicality.

What Type of Exercises Are Good For Natural Childbirth?

An expectant mother wishing to have natural childbirth should first check with her doctor to determine if she seems to be experiencing a normal pregnancy. If the pregnancy is without complications, then usually she is instructed in various exercises that will serve to strengthen and tone the pelvic area.

Hatha Yoga offers exercises that both build the whole body and tone those areas that will be used in the process of child-bearing. It goes without saying that these movements, along with any other exercises, must first be approved by the attending physician, for only he would know if the pregnancy is of such a nature that any undue movement is to be avoided. Where there is approval, then, any and all Yoga exercises that call for flexing and limbering the leg muscles and pelvic area will prove of value.

Deep breathing is of the most vital importance in natural childbirth. It is this practice that will help relieve pain during delivery. The great amount of oxygen supplied by deep-breathing will stabilize the straining body, making the doctor's job easier.

In addition, complete relaxation must be practiced daily in order, when the time comes, for the mother to maintain a completely relaxed body. This in turn will facilitate the birth, and will minimize the chances of any obstruction caused by tautened muscles.

Though all movements of the body will help to prepare it for childbirth, there are some which are particularly valuable. The Squatting exercises help accustom the body to the final position of child-bearing. The Side Leg Stretch, in which the leg is swung out to develop agility of the hip area, is also good preparation.

Sitting in the Easy Pose and the Perfect Pose is an excellent way to stretch the pelvic area. Even more beneficial is the movement recommended when one cannot get one's knee to the floor while attempting these two postures. The gentle bouncing of the knee to the floor in daily practice gradually stretches and flexes the pelvic area in a manner that will bring about the elasticity so needed during childbirth.

Exercises To Be Avoided

In general, all exercises should be of value in any plan to strengthen the body. But because of the variance in body structure, and the differing needs and indispositions of each body, those postures which call for a distinct pull on the abdomen should be avoided in preparing for childbirth.

The Leg Raise and the Bridge are two poses which should be eliminated from an expectant mother's exercise program. Since the Bridge is an excellent back strengthener, it does have great value. However, caution would dictate that other back strengtheners which do not affect the abdominal area be substituted.

As the months advance and birth draws nearer, the body naturally will grow more bulky, at least in the abdominal area. Any awkward body position or movement that might result in a fall must be avoided. This would include the Shoulder Stand and the Head Stand.

Jeanette had grown up on the story of how difficult her birth had been, and how her mother had labored hour after hour until finally the doctor had managed to extract her nine-pound, five-ounce body with his forceps. In fact, the marks of the forceps were so imbedded in her skin that during the first dozen years of her own life whenever she became excited or flushed of face, the faint red marks would be outlined on her forehead and the base of her neck; the points at which the instrument had seized her.

Jeanette determined not to experience a similar birth with her own children. She wanted her children to enter the world naturally; she didn't want birth to be a traumatic experience for them. Nor did she want to contribute any disadvantage to them by being sedated. This would make their struggle for birth greater than necessary. Since she was small of build, just like her mother, she knew she would have to limber every part of her body in order to avoid extreme discomfort during the actual delivery. Her enthusiasm for outdoors activities gave her a good basis on which to commence her childbirth preparations. Because of her natural agility, Jeanette found the practice of Yoga no difficult matter. Avoiding the Plough, and any movement that doubled the abdomen, she practiced all other Yoga exercises to great advantage.

Encountering no difficulties during her pregnancy, Jeanette was free to practice all

PREPARING FOR NATURAL CHILDBIRTH

of the leg stretching and back- and pelvic-strengthening Yoga movements that would prove an invaluable aid during delivery. These movements were as much a part of her day as her carefully planned diet.

Jeanette sailed through the birth of her first child. Her weight gain had been minimal, and her movements during the months of her pregnancy had been easy and unrestricted. There had been no back pain or other physical discomforts during the nine months. She had a quick recovery, and she took home a perfect, healthy child.

With three additional children delivered by natural childbirth, Jeanette feels she can enjoy her children all the more because there are no painful memories attached to their birth.

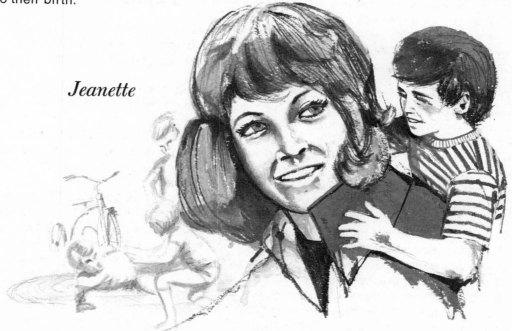

Jeanette

It comes as a surprise to many women who enter a course of study of Yoga to find that in addition to helping themselves in one direction with a specific problem, they have also cleared up another one. There is always great pleasure in finding that in learning to move their body more agilely, they have also eliminated the discomfort that accompanied their menstrual periods.

Arlene was a young woman with a serious monthly problem of almost unbearable pain. Though she worked as a legal secretary in a busy law office, once a month Arlene had to take off that portion of the day when her discomfort commenced. There was an understanding in the office that Arlene "had problems". But her embarrassment wasn't lessened any by the fact that she received silent sympathy from her male employers.

Arlene even considered changing to a job where only a woman would have to be informed of her monthly distress, and she could avoid the acute embarrassment she underwent in her present employment.

Because of the regularity of the problem, Arlene and her mother had a code set up. Arlene, hit with the first cramps presaging worse to come, would call her mother. Then she would excuse herself from the office explaining to her employers that she didn't feel well. Her mother would meanwhile turn down her daughter's bed, fill two hot water bottles and place a glass of gin beside the bed.

Arlene, a teetotaler except for her monthly bouts, would complete this ritual by drinking the gin and preparing for bed, where she would remain for the remainder of the day and night. After a night's sleep, the discomfort lessened enough to permit her to return to work.

This had been the pattern of Arlene's days. She had been told that surgery would correct her problem, but she had delayed going through with this in the hopes that she might overcome the problem in another way.

Recently Arlene had been dieting and had lost weight, but she felt her body was not as firm as it should be. Joining with a friend who had the same objective, she entered a Yoga course with the idea of toning her body in preparation for the summer and a vacation of swimming at a coastal resort.

She responded to the benefits of the stimulating exercises very quickly. She noticed a freshness of feeling that lasted even late into the evening. Her body began to develop tone, and Arlene did not skimp on her preparations for a summertime figure. But her greatest joy came when she noticed an abatement of discomfort the following month during menstruation. Though she did return home, it was more from habit than necessity. For once there, the pains did not increase in intensity, and Arlene found she did not require either the gin or the hot water bottles.

The following month, there was even greater relief. And by the end of the third month of practicing Yoga, Arlene no longer had to leave the office on the day that the cycle began. With no discomfort whatsoever, Arlene was able to continue her usual day without the embarrassment and interruption in her life that had plagued her for so long.

The strengthening of the abdominal area no doubt brought about the welcomed relief. When the body lacks tone, or the inner organs are without elasticity, there is bound to be interference with normal physical functions. With the restoration of elasticity to the body, regular functions can go on unimpeded.

Sally had a similar problem. Being a nurse, she was on her feet during most of the

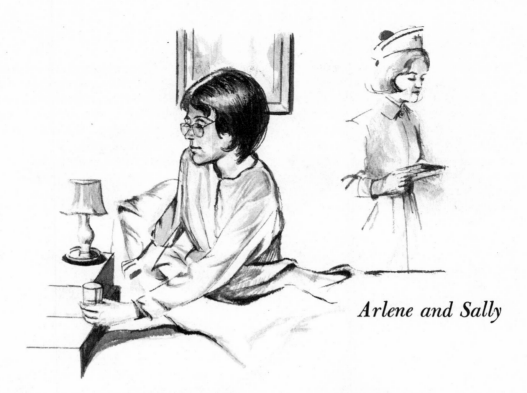

Arlene and Sally

hours of the day. Though efficient and capable, she felt that her own efforts to aid others were hampered by her monthly bouts of discomfort. More times than she cared to admit, she was forced to find a place to rest during the days of her period.

Also, she had begun taking an even stronger drug to ease the pain because the one she had used for years had lost its effectiveness. Sally knew there was codeine in the pills she had to swallow now with increasing frequency, and she resented the fact that even with her knowledge of anatomy, she was so helpless and so reliant on increasingly stronger medicines to bring a measure of relief.

Though she began to practice Yoga because of a desire for more energy in general, she was curious about its effects on her monthly problem. Her problem took longer to clear up than Arlene's, but by the end of four months Sally was no longer on codeine pills. There had been a steady decrease in her monthly discomfort, and with its eventual clearing up and complete correction, Sally turned to her profession with even greater dedication. She is functioning now as a devoted woman, helping others without limitation, because she is not aware of any personal discomfort. Nothing holds her back from the giving that is unique to her profession.

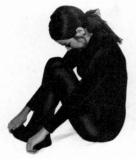
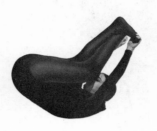
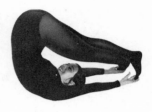

Rocking II

Sit in an Easy Pose, with the legs crossed, and hold onto the left toes with the right hand and the right toes with the left hand. Deep-breathe and rock backward. Straighten the legs as far as they will go in their crossed position, exhale and return to the sitting position. Repeat.

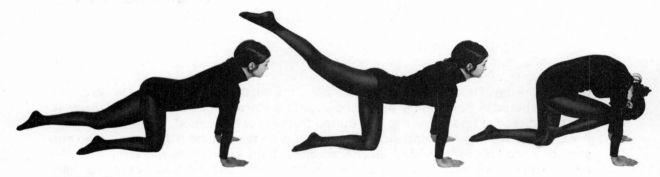

Back Roll

Kneel on the hands and knees so that the back is parallel to the floor. Deep-breathe and raise the right leg into the air, stretching it backward and up until the pull is felt along the spine. Keep the head high. Exhale and bring the leg forward, so that the knee presses against the forehead. Lift the head upward as the knee returns to its position on the floor.

Repeat very slowly several times and then change legs and continue.

It is very helpful to try to roll the spine as the head reaches toward the knee. A rigid and straight spine cannot perform this movement, so the value of consciously assisting the curving of the spine is essential for a completed posture.

PREPARING FOR NATURAL CHILDBIRTH

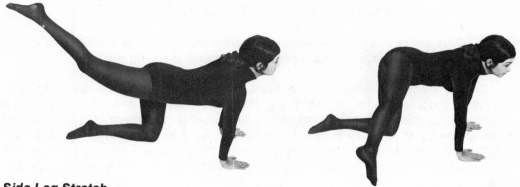

Side Leg Stretch

Kneel on the hands and knees so that the back is parallel to the floor. Deep-breathe and raise the right leg, stretching it backward and up. Keep the head as high as is comfortably possible. Exhale and bring the right leg to the side, keeping the knee perfectly straight. Inhale and return the leg to a straight position behind the body. Exhale and return the leg to a kneeling position. Repeat several times, then reverse the procedure and perform the same exercise with the left leg.

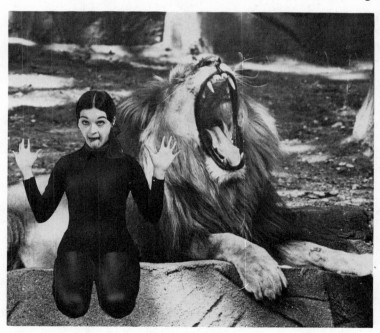

The Lion

Sit on the heels. Place the hands on the knees. Take a deep breath and tense the back. Push the hands out in front and spread the fingers into a stiffened fan shape. Stick the tongue out and downward as far as is possible. Open the eyes as wide as possible and look upward. Tense the entire body during this posture. Exhale with great force and relax. Repeat several times.

EXERCISE BENEFITS IN CHAPTER 6

Rocking II—This second method of rocking produces even greater flexibility of the spine, in addition to adding suppleness to the legs and toning the hips.

Back Roll—The Back Roll affects the entire length of the body when, at its longest line, the posture stretches the body from the head to the toes. Increased suppleness of the vertebrae is gained by the second movement of the Back Roll when the head rolls forward to meet the knee, as it in turn moves forward. The legs and thighs are stretched beneficially as they are brought forward in this firming movement. The buttocks receive a tautening pull that helps to tone the area.

Side Leg Stretch—The Side Leg Stretch works at removing the unattractive "saddle bags" collection of loose flesh that pads the lower area of the hips, and which seems to defy most other body exercises. The buttocks, also a difficult area to exercise effectively, are slimmed down and firmed with daily practice of this movement.

The Lion—The forceful exhalation of the Lion brings blood to the throat for excellent stimulation. Muscles in the throat and the face receive a toning, and in addition, the Lion is considered helpful in preventing colds because it quickens blood circulation to the respiratory tract.

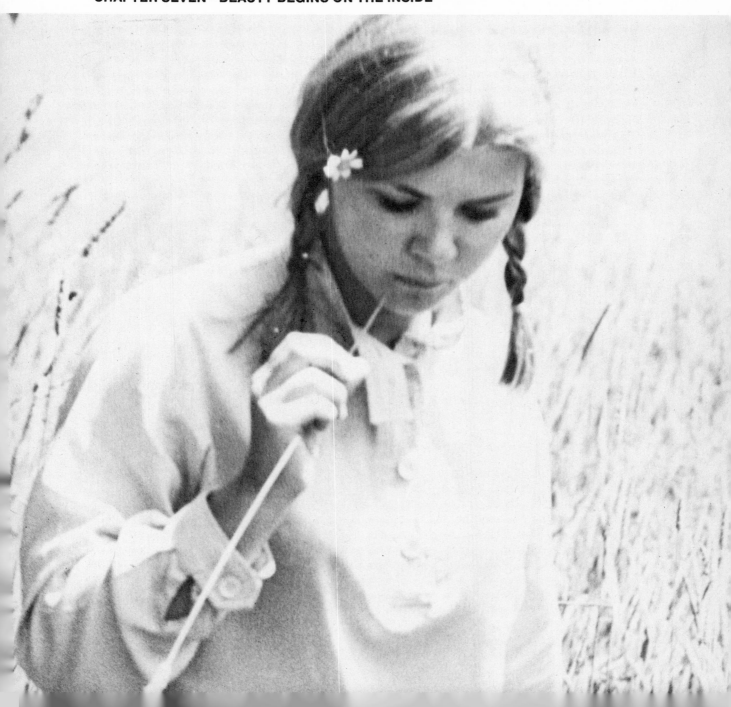

The true elements of beauty are available to all of us, no matter what our physiognomy. Within each body there are the components of life which provide a foundation on which to work. No matter what one's physical structure may be, beauty in one form or another can be developed. In fact, it can be had for the asking, as long as you ask it of yourself, for there must be a sense of dedication and concern in order to bring out the best that exists deep within you.

Because of our concern with outward appearance, the inner person is oft times ignored. And yet it is from this well of great wealth that all natural beauty must come. It is from within that serenity emanates—serenity which smoothes a furrowed brow. Peacefulness of thought will lift a rounded shoulder, straighten a curved back, lift a downward-thrusting chin, and turn lips upward with pleasure. A complexion that has been lathered with creams, annointed with moisturizers, and carefully covered with makeup cannot make up for a deep, negative sag of the muscles.

So all outward contrivances become useless in the pursuit of beauty if that same quality isn't harbored within. This further points up Yoga's lesson that beauty is a quality that must come from practicing self-control and awareness. These qualities will eliminate useless worry and safeguard one against the many assaults of daily living.

Beauty cannot be acquired from an external application alone. Placing a new foundation on the complexion is not going to erase the damage if, within the mind, uncertainties and insecurities fester and push outward in the form of pursed lips, tautened skin, and narrowed eyes that reflect a suspicion of life around one.

Even when there has been a successful restructure of the face by surgical methods, the surgeon warns the recipient of the now-wrinkleless appearance that she must avoid furrowing the face with lines of frustration and worry, if she does not want this new exterior to become the same as the one he corrected.

This means that one is still prey to the same debilitating emotions which produced the premature aging in the first place. If one does not change one's attitude, assuming it is a self-destructive one, it will paint itself across the face in untold lines. Or it may manifest itself in illness that produces the marks of distress on face and figure. In all these cases, the acquisition of a new face by surgery will be a short-lived reprieve.

How much better to commence a rehabilitation of the face and figure by the practice of a discipline that will bring joy *and* beauty, and which cannot vanish with any given year.

In keeping the face free of wrinkles, one does not have to remain expressionless. That sort of appearance would be as bland and as meaningless as the face of a paper doll. But we should understand the error of using our faces to express frequent disapproval, quick anger, annoyance, and other emotional reflections.

Yoga teaches that one must overcome these angers and irritations. Then the face can truly reflect our inner feelings without damage. For the pleasant reflections of comfortable attitudes on the face of a well adjusted and serene woman add interest, rather than age, to her facial lines.

Courage is required to walk the path toward real beauty. Courage to give up previous bad habits that led one to an orgy of rich foods, irregular sleeping hours, and other self-indulgences. Unless one is started on the pathway of health and beauty as a child, and few of us are, it takes a constant marshalling of one's most determined efforts to avoid slipping back into bad habits. But once Yoga exercises are learned, and the results enjoyed, the pathway becomes a marked trail with the destination always only 15 minutes away each day.

Maureen was a handsome woman in her mid-forties. She had always been active in her favorite outdoor sports. Consequently, her body was shapely and well cared for. Because of her brilliant red hair and opaline-type complexion, one's glance went immediately to her face. The view was good. Only one flaw stood out in this well preserved and remarkably youthful appearing woman: a double chin.

When we praise youthfulness, it is not a mere facade we are discussing. It is an attitude; an aliveness that comes from keeping the body and the mind agile. It has nothing to do with wearing too youthful styles and attempting to pass oneself off as younger than one really is. Men and women of 70 can appear youthful if there is a vitality of life about them.

But Maureen's need for a youthful appearance and attitude, was based on necessity. Her position as fashion coordinator for a large department store was constantly threatened by younger, aspiring women. With three children to support and without income other than that from her position, Maureen had to appear at her best, physically, in order to withstand the competition.

Maureen liked her work, and because of her experience and ability, she felt reasonably secure in her position. However, she was distressed over this one aspect of her appearance—her double chin—that suggested she might be self-indulgent. Since Maureen's problem was not medical, but resulted from softened neck muscles which had grown loose and heavy because of lack of exercise, she determined to eliminate this threat to her appearance.

It was the modified Fish that brought her the greatest pleasure in her daily exercising of the neck. She said she could actually feel a pull on the slack skin when she rolled her head backward in this movement to strengthen the neck muscles. Within weeks, Maureen's double chin had disappeared, and in its place was a tautened, youthfully-alive throat of a much younger-appearing woman, to match the rest of her appearance.

Yoga stresses the individuality of each and every person. In general, all bodies respond to all of Yoga. Specifically, one physique may require and respond to a certain posture because of its own specific need. The same exercise, however, may not bring identical rewards to another. This serves to emphasize the distinct difference and needs of each body.

A case in point is Carol. Tall, outgoing in personality, Carol nevertheless felt she had a problem. Flat chests have been in vogue for a while, and the possession of such, by these standards, should not overly concern a young woman. But Carol was unhappy because of her modest chest measurements.

Carol insisted that her concern over her seemingly underdeveloped breasts came from her knowledge of proportions gained as an artist. With her other generous body proportions, Carol felt that her measurements were faulty and she sought out any routine that promised increased chest dimensions. Nor was she defensive when she said she felt it would make her more feminine in appearance.

Carol was like a sleuth on the trail of an exciting clue. She learned to deep-breathe because it would stimulate the body and carry oxygen and nourishment in an enriched bloodstream to all extremities. She learned to perform the Cobra because of its back-strengthening benefits, but she was also on the lookout for the specific exercise which would increase her bust measurements.

When at last she learned the Hand Greeting posture, she was a detective in sight of her quarry. She felt the movement of this posture and knew that her body was receiving the stimulation that would help her physical self to realize its finest tone. This one exercise became Carol's favorite. At any odd moment, her hands would go into the backward stretching position as she inched her hands higher and higher up her back toward her shoulders.

The work involved in learning and practicing the Hand Greeting paid off for Carol. After some months of performing this asana, she announced she had gained one and one-half inches in her bust measurements.

"Now," she said, "I am an aesthetic looking female creature."

With the correct movements used to strengthen the pectoral muscles around the breast area, this part of the body becomes firmer and any tendency toward sagging is eliminated.

Margot's problem was a humiliating one to her. As a successful business woman, she had opened and operated a knit shop. Because of recent requests, she was going to commence giving needlework classes in her shop which would likely increase her sales even further. However, Margot, a skilled needlewoman, could not wear the creations she could make and could teach others to make.

Her embarrassment was acute, for she did not dare to appear in the clinging knitted dresses. In her drive to establish herself in business, Margot had neglected herself over a period of several years. The results were thickly-padded buttocks and heavy thighs, all

BEAUTY BEGINS ON THE INSIDE

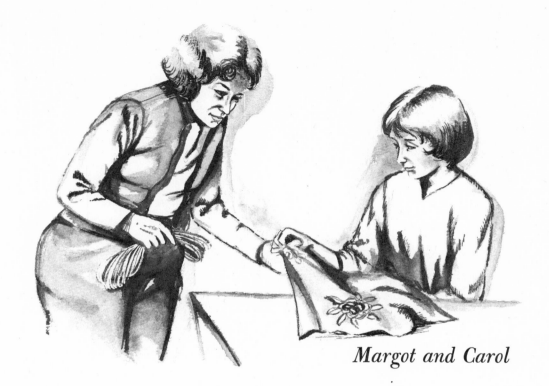

Margot and Carol

of which would be emphasized in a knitted fabric.

Margot applied herself to Yoga just as she had done making a success of her business. On the day that she began to practice the beginning exercises, she methodically listed all her body measurements and put the information aside. Each day she performed the various asanas and each week she would learn new ones to add to her previous ones. There were the beginning asanas that dealt with the spine, the neck, and the abdomen that had to be learned first.

By the time the Leg Stretch and the Side Leg Stretch appeared in her lessons, Margot's body was supple enough to perform toning and whittling exercises easily.

It was not long before the sagging buttocks area firmed up and with this transformation, Margot's thighs began to lose their saddlebag appearance. The huge bulges that had created a too full-blown caricature of Margot's figure disappeared. Her delight in her new appearance led her to create a flattering knit dress for herself. Her pleasure was heightened when students in her knitting class asked to have the pattern made available to them.

While improving the figure is always desirable, Yoga works in other ways as well. With the physical change in Margot's measurements, a change in her mental attitude also developed. With the removal of excess flesh that speaks of self-indulgence, lack of will power, or indifference, goes also the defensive attitudes one develops. So it was that Margot became a more agreeable and pleasant person, because she had acquired a reasonable pride in learning to control her body.

For one who is sensitive, there is always the probable damage to the ego when the body proportions are at a great variance with accepted norms. Much time is spent excusing, apologizing, or defending one's imperfect appearance.

Yoga teaches that one should develop the discipline that will lead to avoidance of irritants or excesses to the body, while at the same time, learning to live at peace with the physique that has limitations about which nothing can be done.

While bringing the body to its highest personal performance, the mind is learning the discipline of serenity. And no matter at what point a personal limit in physical achievement is reached, this serenity will continue to grow.

Debbie's automobile accident had damaged her body to the extent that she distrusted unnecessary physical movement. As a consequence, this lovely girl further damaged her rigid back by permitting it no exercise that would gain her a degree of flexibility.

Increasing discomfort came from a bend to retrieve a fallen object. Debbie even resisted a desire to yawn, for so stiffened had her spinal column become that stretching in any direction brought sharp aches to the back area.

No more outdoor activities, no more youthful romps; moreover, a deep frown was developing across this pretty girl's forehead. Living grew increasingly limited, and the consequences of a narrowed life style had removed much of the spontaneous beauty that had chased across Debbie's face. Discomfort and quick displeasure etched deep vertical lines around her lips. Her weakened spine no longer was the basis of a beautiful carriage, and in consequence, Debbie developed an unattractive slump to her shoulders. But Debbie mentally shrugged and accepted this as the inevitable result of her accident. She tried to learn to live with this disability. But life was becoming tiresome.

When Debbie finally decided she could not continue to function as a half-alive person, she turned to Yoga as a means of regaining the use of her body.

One day Debbie read about a woman, twice her age, who had overcome far greater disabilities than her own. The woman had suffered through years in a concentration camp and survived, only to find herself, in later years, caught in a burning building from which her only escape lay in jumping from an upper window. Though the woman escaped with her life, she was left with a body so badly hurt by the fall that she suffered pain for years, without any relief, until she began to practice Yoga.

BEAUTY BEGINS ON THE INSIDE

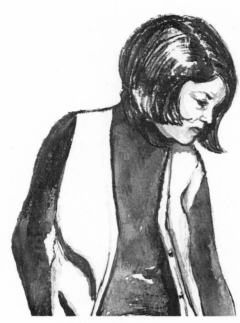

Debbie and Betsy

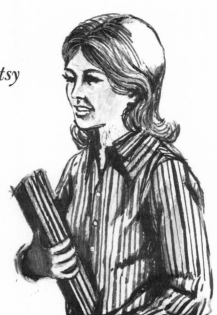

The story was an inspiration to Debbie, for she learned that the woman had not only overcome her own disabilities, but actually began to teach Yoga after her recovery, and enjoyed a pain-free and beautifully resurrected body.

With this story in mind, Debbie began to practice Yoga. In the beginning she was hardly more than a spectator. While others were involved in learning the Plough and advancing on into the Headstand, Debbie was learning to roll her body into a ball in an attempt to achieve a more supple spine.

Yoga suggests that every one advance at his own rate of speed, and this was Debbie's. As long as the body is kept moving, one can advance. It does not matter at what rate of speed it comes, for advancement is sometimes a thing of the spirit. Debbie knew that she was being helped by her careful movements, and this was enough for the moment.

Her slow approach was rewarding. Very conscious of her rigid spine, she did not force her body into a position. When she advanced from her first posture to another, she would not perform the posture more than once daily until she felt it was comfortable to do so. In time she advanced to the posture of the Plough. Her legs remained suspended in mid-air week after week, instead of touching the floor behind her head. But this was not important. Debbie was moving her spine, and the improvement over her condition many weeks earlier was impressive.

Debbie regained the full use of her spine. Today she can do the Shoulder Stand with the ease of an agile person. Her spinal column offers no opposition to the Plough position. Debbie feels she appreciates her body and its wonderful abilities all the more because she has come so far from the almost invalid existence of earlier months.

Betsy was a sleepy-eyed young nineteen-year-old when she attended her first class of Yoga. It was, she said, a last resort. She'd tried just about everything she'd ever known that was supposed to give one energy. Betsy was a college sophomore who knew she had to make the most of every year of her education. She planned a medical career, and the long years lying ahead would require much financial sacrifice on the part of her family.

Betsy's problem was fatigue, for in addition to her studies, she had a part-time job. She had tried all the popular pep pills used by students and by truck drivers who force themselves to function on highways long after their bodies rebel from lack of sleep. Pep pills, bennies, and other amphetamines were some of the stimulants Betsy had used in an effort to get through her long classes and lectures, and in order to spend her late evenings studying.

But the various pep pills had a drawback. When she relied on the artificial stimulants to keep her going, Betsy had to take depressants in order to sleep, even after a long day. Otherwise, she would lie in bed and find dawn coming up without having had adequate sleep throughout the night.

Driven by a sense of responsibility and a genuine desire for an education, Betsy was carrying a heavy program. But she could succeed, she felt, if she could find the energy to carry her studies and her part-time job too. Lately she found herself dozing at lectures, and even at work.

Betsy's problem was not a complicated one, nor even one that was difficult to meet. This ambitious young woman was so busy preparing for the future she was not adequately serving the present needs of her body. Before one can successfully operate under a heavy work schedule, one must first get into the finest physical condition. This means mastering deep-breathing exercises, learning to relax and moving all the parts of the body in a beneficial way to keep blood flowing and to avoid sluggishness.

Betsy learned to employ deep-breathing and the Yoga Mudra as a stimulator before classes. This rejuvenating asana brings blood to the brain, as it simultaneously relaxes a tense body. Betsy needed all the health-giving Yogic movements. But she especially needed the freshened blood supply to stay alert.

Before any class, if she felt a sense of lethargy, Betsy would find an open window or door. Slowly, with deep breathing, she would lift her arms upward as she dipped her head downward to a point that she could feel the blood surging through her face.

Did anyone think it strange to see her employing Yogic movements on the campus? Not at all. In fact, when friends saw the change that came over the formerly somnambulant Betsy, there were more than a few converts to Betsy's program of rejuvenation.

BEAUTY BEGINS ON THE INSIDE

Hand Greeting

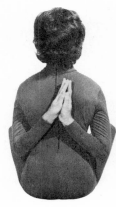

Sit in a cross-legged position on the floor. Hold the spine straight and bring the arms around to the back. Place the palms together at the lower portion of the back, avoiding any strain. While deep-breathing in and out, slowly bring the palms up the back as high as possible. Keep the palms together. Remember to keep the back straight and to avoid the tendency to roll the shoulders forward as the attempt is made to reach higher with the hands.

As facility is gained in reaching a certain height, work upward again, but do not push or force the arms unwillingly upward.

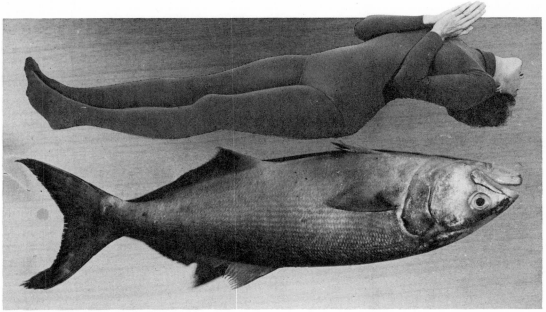

Modified Fish

Lie flat on the floor on the back. Deep-breathe and slowly roll the head back until the shoulders leave the floor. Bring the palms together over the chest with the elbows lifted from the floor. The weight should be felt on the head and the buttocks.

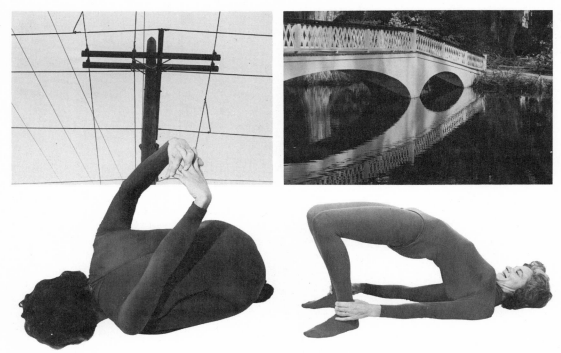

Yoga Mudra

The word Mudra refers to the ability to create a vital current by a particular pose of the limbs. This is one of many Mudras.

In a kneeling position, with the buttocks on the heels, and with the hands clasped behind the back, deep-breathe, exhale, and bring the head down to the floor. Do not permit the buttocks to leave the heels. With the head touching the floor, the arms will be held straight over the head. Inhale and come up. Relax and repeat.

The Bridge

Lie flat on the floor, on the back, with the arms lying comfortably by the sides. Raise the knees upward so that the heels are close to the buttocks. Grasp the ankles with the hands. Deep-breathe and bring the buttocks off the floor until all the weight of the body is concentrated on the shoulders and the arms. Exhale and come down.

While it is easier for some to first manage this position with the legs widely separated, the legs should be brought closer together with practice.

EXERCISE BENEFITS IN CHAPTER 7

Hand Greeting—This posture encourages greater movement and control of the shoulders as it exercises, by pull, the entire chest area. The pectoral muscles are also strengthened.

The Modified Fish—Practiced slowly, the Fish stretches the neck and upper cervical area. It also stimulates the thyroid gland and is effective against respiratory complaints.

The Yoga Mudra—This asana is a symbol of Yoga. In our Westernized version, we kneel and proceed with the original Yoga Mudra movement which lifts the arms overhead in a stretching action. While it has a tranquilizing effect on the body and the mind, it is also used for toning a bulging waistline. In addition, the entire pelvic area benefits from this stimulating activity.

The Bridge—The Bridge produces muscle tone for the abdominal area even as it increases spinal suppleness. By bending the back in an opposite direction to the usual forward bend, the inward curving gives a more effective spinal exercise. It is a back-strengthener, but one to be approached with caution by anyone with a back ailment.

Because of the arched position of the stomach as this area is raised upward, the Bridge is considered an excellent exercise for strengthening the stomach.

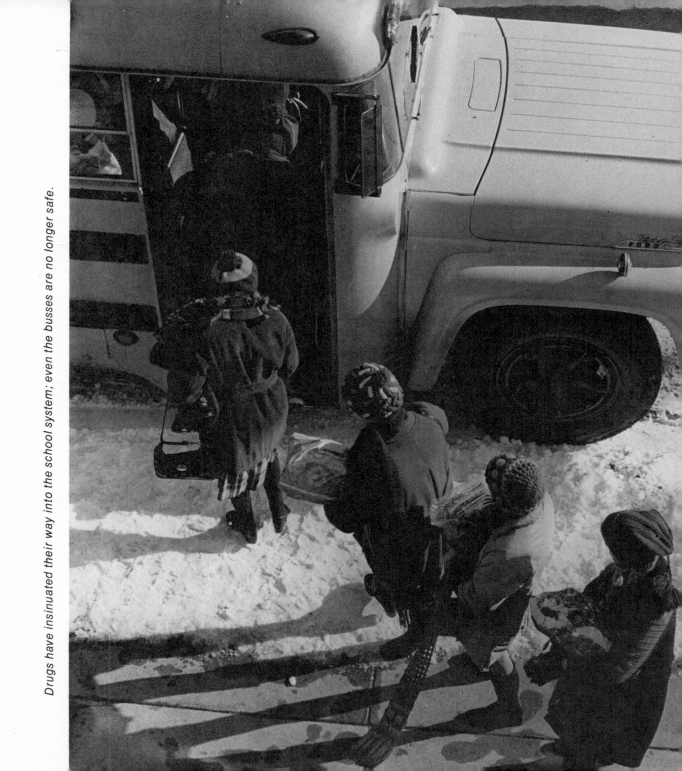

Drugs have insinuated their way into the school system; even the busses are no longer safe.

CHAPTER EIGHT - THEY FOUGHT DRUGS ---- AND WON

Drug usage had hit the local high school. It hadn't come suddenly, nor was there just a recent awareness of this problem. But usage had reached danger proportions, involving a major percentage of the two upper classes, and the problem could no longer be dealt with on an individual basis.

No longer could Johnny or Susie be brought, with their parents, before the principal and the situation discussed, the student dismissed, and the school cleared of a major distress. In order to do this, to clear away the drug problem by this method, an estimated 70% of the two upper classes would have to be expelled. These were alarming proportions. For a while, lectures on the subject seemed to be helping. There was even a proposal to take the students to a facility where brain-damaged drug addicts were treated.

It was decided to have a representative from this nearby institution come and address the student body on the ills of drug addiction. While this presentation no doubt deterred some students from the dangerous involvement, those already habituated continued their usage.

The School Board grew desperate. They knew the next step, if the drug taking was not stopped, or at least lessened to a manageable degree, would be a complete loss of control of their students.

Various methods for dealing with the problem that has become a national scourge were discussed.

Yoga was proposed as a means of teaching youngsters to care for their bodies, to awaken them to the value of self-control when all around them self-discipline was falling away.

With Yoga accepted as a possible deterrent to drug usage, arrangements were made to secure a teacher knowledgeable in the chemistry of drugs, the pitfalls of addiction, and the practice of Yoga.

Special emphasis was to be placed on the aspect of self-discipline. Nutrition would also be a part of the course, with suggestions that many of the sweets consumed in such large amounts, and suspected of bringing about instability in the human mind, be replaced with unrefined products. An attempt would be made to guide the students into an awareness of the role nutrition and regular exercise play in molding their attitudes toward life and the use of drugs.

But in large part, the Yoga course would attempt to awaken interest in developing and maintaining a beautiful body and a serene mind capable of coping with the problems of youth. Pride in the masterful design of the body would be stressed, hopefully warding off the temptation to indulge in drugs that would destroy the body by attacking the mind.

It was agreed that emphasis would not be placed on drug usage itself, for fear of turning off the students' interest. The assets and positiveness of Yoga were to be emphasized, instead.

This was easy to do, for Yoga—itself a moderate practice—could speak simply and fittingly of any aspect of the body and mind. By nature a positive approach to life, Yoga would help to open up formerly negative areas of the students' thoughts.

The teacher selected for leading a group of the students into the practice of Hatha Yoga was herself the mother of three teenagers. And as such, she was aware of the problems all too prevalent in the schools.

She was able to point out that the so-called mind-expansion drugs were in fact mind-stultifying, and destructive in their artificial stimulation. She approached the class with a calm that came from her long association with Yogic practices. Curiosity, diffidence, and a frequent "show me" attitude greeted her in the classroom.

Concentrating on movements needed to develop a healthy body, and deep breathing techniques intended to cleanse the lungs and give the body more oxygen, Joy Gorin spoke also of the ability of oxygen in sufficient quantity to control some types of irrational behavior.

She had worked with mentally disturbed children in various clinics, teaching them Yoga postures, and her reward had been a breakthrough in contact with otherwise non-communicative youngsters. She credited this in part to the increased oxygen supply to the body and mind.

The majority of youngsters in her teenage class at the high school had tried one or more drugs, and probably would have continued with their destructive experimenting. But this Yoga teacher was effective in her work. She taught the students how to achieve the same feeling of relaxation, release, and mind-expansion from Yoga exercises that they had found in drug-taking. The difference was in the fact that there were no harmful side effects from Yoga practices; only a growing awareness of the potential of the human body and mind when they are kept in a natural condition and not assaulted with artificial stimulants.

True mind expansion cannot come from an artificial source. The use of drugs is a form

THEY FOUGHT DRUGS ---- AND WON

of distortion, and cannot be compared with the great sense of release from petty emotions and even seriously discordant ones, gained by practicing Yoga. For only the healthy mind and body are capable of complete happiness.

Drug usage dropped in this group. Students taking the course discovered that their bodies and minds were capable of creating all of the escape or accomplishment they needed. Pride began to develop in previously indifferent students.

Now, with the demonstrated success of Yoga practices in curbing undisciplined use of drugs, more and more young people are turning to this discipline as a way of living that can enhance, rather than destroy, their lives.

Teen drug usage finds its adult counterpart of destruction in alcoholism. The latter problem is one of longer standing, but of equal concern, because it seems many unstable individuals who escape drug addiction have the potential of succumbing, later in life, to the addiction of alcohol.

Sanatoria dedicated to the treatment and prevention of alcoholism have tried many and varying treatments in their approach to this now world-wide problem. Some methods have been successful, others have not. It would seem that a dislike for one's own person would make one particularly vulnerable to alcohol. In an attempt to escape, one turns to this method of dulling the senses, so as not to be as aware of oneself, therefore, not so conscious of personal dislike.

Yoga stresses the need to know and like oneself, in order to overcome weaknesses, if they exist. Where there is a definite problem, then a direct attack upon its cause and an attempt to correct its practice should eliminate any need to escape.

Karen came to her first Yoga class with her problem, or the effects of it, in plain evidence. Bright-eyed and unnaturally flushed of face, she owed her present degree of comfort to several drinks she had had.

Karen had been trying to drink away her problem of being married to an ambitious young man who wanted more from life than a nine-to-five job, and a companionable evening alone with his wife.

Karen's family had been close. Brothers and sisters and parents formed a well-knit family circle, sufficient unto themselves, and needing no outsiders, as they said. From this virtually closed life of affection and attention, Karen married an out-of-state young man whose family lived in yet another part of the country.

Alone in a large city with too much time to herself and no real organization to her days, Karen resented the hectic pace that their lives had assumed because of her husband's determination to rise swiftly to a prominent position in his law firm. At first rebelling against the frequent partying that their new status dictated, Karen avoided the cocktail table and bar. She spent many hours holding onto a glass of fruit juice during the first year of her marriage.

Gradually Karen discovered that the functions grew less long and less boring if she had a drink. If she had two, the people began to appear less foolish in their constant chatter. As she worked up the scale toward alcoholism, Karen tried to convince herself this was not of her doing, that her husband chose this kind of life, therefore, let him suffer the consequences of her drinking.

Gradually the cocktail hour moved backward in the day until she began her drinking at noon as she lunched with wives of her husband's colleagues. Karen was a casual drinker only a short time before she progressed to the role of a serious drinker. Her husband finally noticed what was happening.

There were trips to a psychiatrist, and extended visits to a clinic which encouraged withdrawal from alcohol. But once she returned to her pattern of life with her husband, Karen again drifted into the same drinking habits. One of her husband's colleagues introduced her to Yoga. He said it was his belief that the wife of every professional man, whose career depended in great measure on his ability to mix with people and form important new contacts, should be introduced to the practice of Yoga as soon as the honeymoon was over.

Yoga helps in so many aspects of living that it is not surprising it can offer aid to the woman who, for her husband's sake, is under constant pressure to live a publicly social life.

Karen had to understand that her hus-

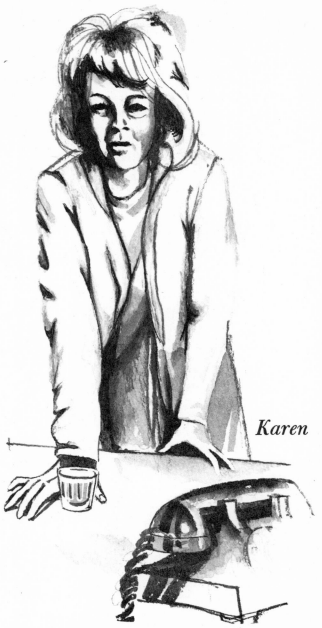

Karen

THEY FOUGHT DRUGS ---- AND WON

band would never be happy with the singularly uncomplicated life she preferred. Nor had she a right to deny him his ambitions. If she chose not to help him, that was one thing. But to blame him for her own resentments and disappointments and to exact a payment in concern was the act of an immature person.

Karen arrived at the first two or three of her classes with the strong alcohol odor which had become a part of her entrance wherever she went. As she rolled backward and forward she giggled helplessly. But no one disturbed her with stares, for a Yoga class is an unusually heartwarming place. The students are people in search of many and varied destinations and goals. There is always pleasure when they see a member achieve some difficult and long sought-after position, but there is no idle curiosity.

Yoga practitioners could be compared to the goldminers panning a stream for nuggets of the precious metal. While they may show increased hope when a fellow panner reveals the gleaming metal in his basket, the miner knows it is not until *he* sees gold in his own pan that he is successful. And the complete absence of the searched-for gold leaves the searcher uninterested in anything other than this striving for his own goal.

The lesser emotions of envy and scorn either do not belong to those who practice Yoga, or else are soon discarded along with other debilitating attitudes.

With this accepting and pleasant atmosphere around her, Karen did not avoid coming to class because of her drinking. Admittedly, her drinking didn't stop abruptly. She did not suddenly appear sober and make everyone aware that she had solved her problem. It was more involved than an instant cure. Again, one might compare this awareness with the attitude necessary to bring about a sustained weight loss. Many so-called wonder diets will work, if the only problem is to lose weight quickly. But we know from experience that only a change in thinking will bring about a permanent and desirable change in a weight problem. Otherwise, once the goal of a specified number of pounds is achieved, unless the erroneous thinking that led to the problem is explored, understood, and corrected, the tendency is to return to old eating patterns.

In the same way, it is necessary to understand the problem that led to drinking. Had Karen really liked herself in the first place, she could not have indulged in such a destructive habit.

She explored this thought in Yoga. She was taught relaxation and concentration; she studied the various philosophies that spoke of knowing and liking oneself enough not to harm oneself in any manner.

Karen struggled with her problem of excess drinking, but she was not foolish enough to fail to see her present path of self-destruction. So she concentrated on learning to like herself. She also found the Woodchopper to be especially helpful in its thoroughly relaxing movements. The cleansing of the lungs by the long-expelled breath gave her a feeling of rejuvenation. A chance, she said, of beginning again with each new breath.

She used deep breathing with her exercises and learned to employ this technique as a means of resisting the temptation to drink. The extra intake of oxygen at a moment of weakness and indecision served to give a feeling of buoyancy, a quality which she previously had associated with alcohol.

Karen continues to use her Yoga practices as a means of discipline and growth. But the discipline has turned her back into the non-drinker of earlier years with the additional benefit of making her more aware of herself as a person. Today she works as a partner with her husband and has learned to become a more flexible person, instead of one so tuned in to her needs that she could not part with the customs of an earlier life.

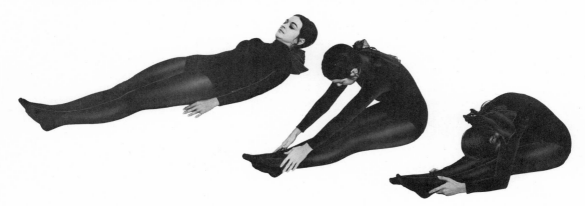

Head to Knee II

Lie flat on the floor on the back. Taking a deep breath, inhale and come to a sitting position. Exhale as you bring the head toward the knee. At the same time, bring the arms and the elbows to the floor as you reach for your feet. Continue to deep breathe, and on the inhale return to a sitting position. On exhale return to a prone position on the floor with your arms by your side.

The Wood Chopper (illustrated on right)

Stand with the feet apart. Clasp the hands together and interlock the fingers. Deep breathe and bring the arms over the head. Roll the spine back as far as it will comfortably go. Imagine that you are holding a very heavy axe in your hands. Open your mouth and exhale heavily through it and bring your arms down, as if you were chopping a log. Bend at the waist and push as much breath out as possible as you exhale.

THEY FOUGHT DRUGS ---- AND WON

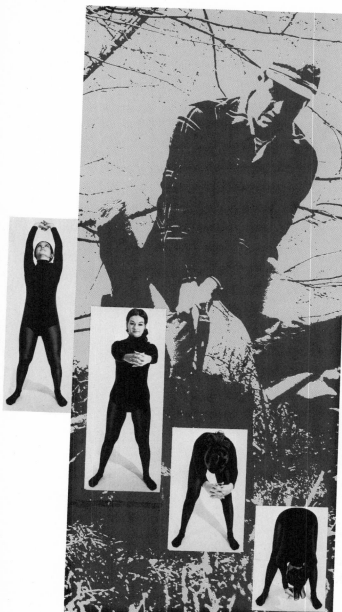

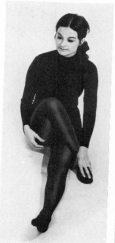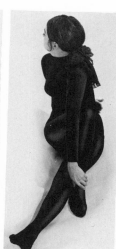

The Twist

Place both feet straight before you as you sit on the floor. Bring the right foot over the left knee, with the sole of that foot placed flat on the floor. Bring the left arm around to the right of the right knee and grasp the ankle of the right foot. Place the right arm around the waistline of the back of the body with the open palm pointing outward. Hold the spine upright. Deep breathe during the posture, and exhale as you slowly turn toward the right. Continue to deep breathe as you hold the position, and exhale as you slowly return to a straight position.

Leave the position very slowly, first returning the head and shoulders to front and center. Relax your left arm and remove it from its position. Return the right leg to its prone position outstretched before you. Relax.

LOOK YOUNGER - LOOK PRETTIER

Reverse all positions by using the left leg, the right arm around the left leg, the left arm around the waist behind you, and by turning the head and shoulders toward the left. Deep breathe in and out.

The Locust

Lying flat on the floor on the stomach, place the fists under the groin. Keep the chin on the floor. Taking a deep breath, raise both legs as far as you comfortably can without any strain. Exhale and come down.

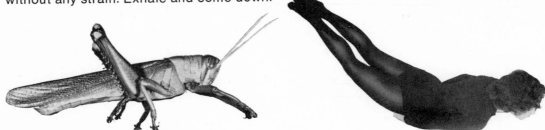

EXERCISE BENEFITS IN CHAPTER 8

Head to Knee II—The second Head-to-Knee posture is a continuation in toning the body. This pose is helpful in relieving indigestion and in activating lazy bowels. Because of the rounded movement of the back when the arms reach for the feet, there is a strengthening effect of the entire back.

The Wood Chopper—Elasticity is brought to the waist by the repeated downward swinging movements of this stimulating exercise. The spine is brought into a limber state and the accumulated toxins resulting from the effects of shallow breathing can be disposed of by the deliberately strong exhalations.

The Twist—This spiraling type of movement presents the picture of a difficult pose. And yet, taken in slow steps, it is easily accomplished. Problems of indigestion can be overcome by the Twist, and the internal organs receive a gentle toning by its practice. It is also helpful in slimming down ungainly thighs.

Locust—This completed posture can be used to tone weakened abdominal muscles. The spine receives an inward curving as both legs are brought up into the air. Caution is to be exercised here in avoiding any strain while attempting this position. The Locust is also considered an aid in strengthening the sex glands.

THEY FOUGHT DRUGS ---- AND WON

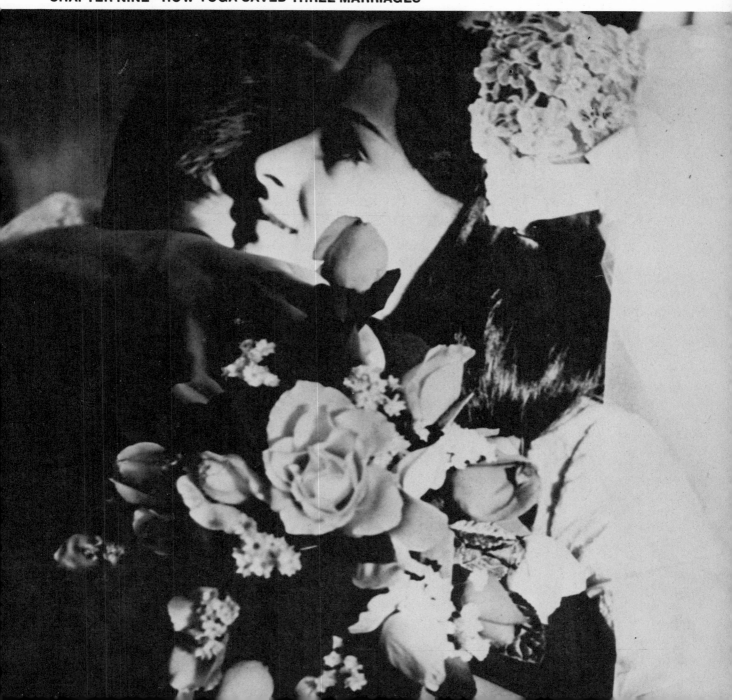

Except for a quirk of fate, some lives would be lived out on a make-do basis. Adjustments are made to uncomfortable situations, and many times the most meaningful summary of the years shared by two people in marriage is "They made do."

In itself, this is an unfortunate waste of lives. No one in a situation that can be changed for the better should be commended for making do, or getting by. The loss of opportunities in living is too overwhelming to calculate.

While Yoga does not hold itself to be a healer of breaches, or a patcher of broken marriages, it has, in fact, performed just such miracles. But never in the sense of entering the fray and deciding rights and wrongs. Yoga does not concern itself with arbitration. Rather, this discipline teaches one the value of knowing oneself and working toward developing the finer qualities. It awakens sluggish bodies and helps to dispose of senseless antipathy toward others.

How is this accomplished? The first step is in the first lesson. The second step is in the second lesson. By following the simple, believable routine of exercising the body and correcting physical distresses and discomforts, the mind is permitted once again to free itself from destructive thoughts, malicious intents, and petty attitudes. In this manner, the mind can rise so far above dissension that sympathy and understanding for another often can solve one's own dilemmas.

Destructive thoughts will eventually affect the physical body. If no mental restraint is practiced, in time the turbulent and festering emotions aroused by one's dislike of another will lead either to development of an unpleasant personality, or if bottled up, to actual physical distresses.

To free oneself from an intolerable situation, one's first step is to free the mind. Knowledge of oneself leads to this.

One couple seemed to live in anticipation of their summer vacation. As soon as their youngsters were out of school, Laura headed for another state where her family lived. Her bags and theirs were packed and waiting long before departure time. Picking her children up at school that last day, Laura would head south, scarcely stopping until she arrived at her destination, so eager was she to put distance between her husband and herself.

Back in their own city, her husband would feel a sense of freedom in his wife's departure. He would make extensive plans for weekends of fishing, travelling around locally, and once he even decided he would visit Europe. These were the kinds of vacations this once happy couple now desired. Separate vacations to match their separate lives.

They had both lost touch with each other years earlier. Laura considered they were mismatched, and her husband felt he had erred in judgment in marrying Laura. The truth

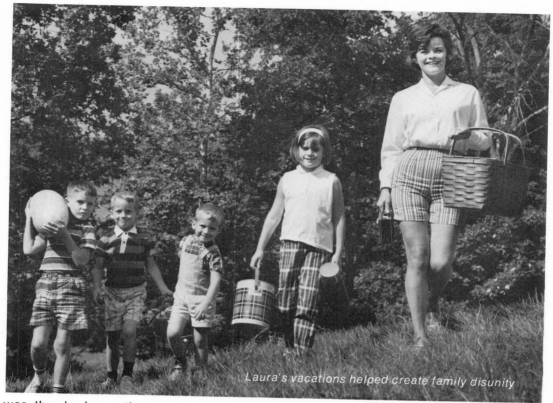

Laura's vacations helped create family disunity

was, they had no estimate of the value of a good marriage, nor the incredible rewards of a marriage that was lovingly guarded and looked over, as one would tend any growing thing. After the first pleasures lessened, they both turned away from each other, as though from a deceiving individual.

As Laura withdrew, her husband shrugged and applied himself to his work, which did not offer such a perplexing challenge as his marriage. Laura decided marriage wasn't all she had thought it to be, and stung by her husband's casual indifference, she busied herself with anything that did not involve him. And there were always the three summer months when they knew they would be apart, plus Christmas and various other times during the school year when a vacation could be fitted in.

But the business in which Laura's husband was engaged failed, and he found himself struggling to hold onto his abbreviated income.

LOOK YOUNGER - LOOK PRETTIER

"We don't really like each other," said Laura. "But then, there are the children. Mentally, I pack my bags several times a day all year around. But to be honest, I'm exhausted from all this stationary running."

During the summer, which she now had to spend at home, Laura tried to fill her hours with new interests. Finding herself in a Yoga class with a group of friends, Laura was completely at ease.

"It was like an introduction to living," she said after a few weeks of practicing daily exercises. "I don't think I've ever been completely alive. No wonder my marriage has failed. I marvel that it could even have made it as far as this."

Laura's underactive days had produced a stagnant attitude in her. That she owed a debt to life for living had never occurred to her. She began to notice people around her more distinctly. Sights, sounds, and the aroma of life became a heady brew. There was so much to make up for.

There was her marriage. Laura grew cautious here. She did her work through the children. An impromptu outing was planned and her husband went along with them. In all their years together with their children, they had never developed a unity of family feeling. Laura had seen no reason for this. The less she saw of her husband, previously, the better she thought she felt.

Slowly, combining her increased awareness of self and the world around her, Laura made headway. Her husband did not object to the company and attention of a pleasant woman. Laura learned to listen, to be sympathetic, and most of all, Laura learned to be an adult involved with another adult in a relationship that, though fragile, had survived damaging treatment. As Laura developed into a more stimulated person, she became aware of the hollowness of their marriage, of the waste and uselessness of their lives together.

Bit by bit Laura chipped away at the indifference that had grown between them. In his turn, her husband acknowledged her efforts and helped to restore to their marriage the life that had been missing for so long.

Laura has not relinquished her exercises. They had aroused a sleeping woman and helped her to awaken a drowsing man. In particular, she practices the Cat, for this stimulation of the abdominal area is an excellent exercise for the gonads, or sex glands. As these glands are rejuvenated, they help to create a radiance and glow of life in the person affected.

Many men and women, practicing Yoga during their middle years, are pleasantly surprised at the rekindled emotions they experience, as these glands are stimulated. Resurgence of glandular activity extends to many areas of the body - the general tone-up brings vitality that disappeared with youth.

More than one woman has had a second chance at her marriage because of the life-force awakened in a sluggish body that had never before been able to respond. And many women have found it possible to return affectionate overtures to husbands who had known only a passive marriage in the past.

In other marriages, a malfunctioning body created by lack of physical exercise and an overrich diet can erase even the earlier memories of happiness.

Joyce's chubby figure was bulging in her leotards. She announced firmly, that first evening in class, that she had no intention of remaining this way. With that she embarked on a self-improvement course. She had carefully planned her activity for the next ten weeks. By the time she had practiced Yoga for this length of time, she assured those around her, they would see a new woman.

Many people will commence laudable efforts of self-improvement with frenzied rather than dedicated attitudes. Yoga, practiced faithfully day by day, will help remove those traits that lead to such emotional declarations in the first place.

It had taken a major upheaval in Joyce's personal life—she was in her early fifties—to spur her to reclaim her body from its padded covering of superfluous fat.

Her husband was having an affair. She accepted this as something that a husband might do, and something a wife could accept and preserve her marriage, or reject and find herself alone. But it didn't work this way for her. Though she unhappily accepted the evidence of the liaison, she was not prepared for the fact that her husband would decide he no longer cared to remain with her.

Joyce suffered shock over her husband's proposal that a divorce would be the solution to their rather indifferent marriage. She fought for time and answers. What had happened to the marriage that had given them such pleasure and closeness during the earlier years? What had caused this hiatus that might put them on the opposite sides of a courtroom?

Joyce knew that she was largely to blame. Her husband had retained his litheness of body to a surprising degree. He had also pursued his work and the varied interests of a man with a questing, curious mind. He had continued to grow mentally while Joyce had ceased most of her mental activity when their first child was born. She had remained the same charming and helpful person she had been twenty years earlier. Except, at that point in life, those two qualities seemed enough for her. They had gotten her a husband and a family. Beyond that she had no aspirations. No desire to know anything of the world around her, if it did not touch directly on her own life, or those nearest her.

With her desires thus limited, Joyce enjoyed nothing more than lining the pantry shelves with glistening jars of preserves and baking a double rich chocolate cake to have with afternoon tea. And in later years, a huge pan of fudge, to have on hand in case the grandchildren should stop by.

There was no stimulation. Joyce was a pleasant, bland woman who had wrapped her-

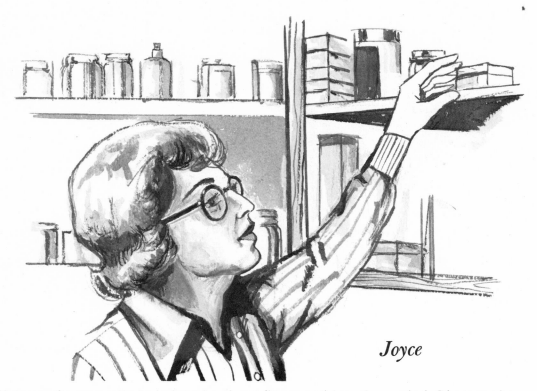

Joyce

self into a soft cocoon that produced a plump figure and incurious mind. Of course her husband lost interest in her. In his business world, he daily was in contact with women who had all the qualities of his own wife, plus the additional benefits of a stimulating personality, and an attractive physical appearance. When he returned home each evening, it was to a sameness of living that never varied, never offered satisfaction to an active mind. There was not even any physical beauty in the woman who had remained on the same mental level as the day he married her. The changes had all been physical; Joyce's acquisition of extra weight exacted a toll, dulling both body and mind.

With her husband's proposal to dissolve their twenty-five-year-old marriage. Joyce was shocked into action. She bargained. Give me time, she asked. Allow me to try to correct all these faults which I never recognized as such. Give me a chance to become a person instead of continuing on this level for the rest of my life, which I probably would do if there is no second chance.

Her husband agreed, though he doubted that after so many years, during which she had never had such an inclination, she could now actually do anything about her pathetic condition. Perhaps she could lose a few pounds. But their discussion and bargain called for a completely changed person; no more days spent in the kitchen preparing meals too ornate and rich for anyone, especially people their age; or days spent in useless squander, accomplishing nothing, profiting no one and giving no pleasure, just getting through a day until time for another meal, or tea, or a snack.

Joyce agreed to it all, and turned to Yoga to help shed pounds and widen her horizons. She struggled with every posture. At times utter defeat would stalk her face. But after a moment's indulgence, she would be back again, working at the posture, or if it proved beyond her, she would simply roll herself into a ball and rock and roll until she felt a limberness. She would remember that this was a proving ground for her, and one of her own choice.

Practicing the physical exercise was not the only part of Joyce's campaign. She took notes on nutrition, locked away her cake pans, and cancelled deliveries of coffee, cream and heavy whipping cream. Grams of protein were counted, and carbohydrates were carefully watched. White sugar and flour disappeared from her kitchen. Accumulated soft drink bottles were returned, deposits received and a vegetable juicer was installed where the mixmaster had stood on her kitchen counter.

Joyce exchanged recipes with other Yoga students—everthing from cranberry juice cocktails to new ways of serving broiled chicken. She learned to carry a handful of sunflower seeds in her pocket for an energy snack, instead of reaching for a piece of candy.

The next step was registration for a course of study at the local college. She looked for areas of awakened interest created by her recent rediscovery of the world around her.

The combination of exercise, dieting, improved nutrition, and exposure to the stimulating thought in the youthful college atmosphere began to have an effect. Joyce steadily shed her obese poundage. She developed a glow from her improved nutrition and a manner of walking far different from her earlier shuffling gait.

She became so busy in her quest to feel even more alive, that her fears about losing her husband lessened. She became, in her words, a woman in pursuit of herself, rather than a woman in pursuit of her husband. Because of the almost unbelievable change he saw in this woman who, for twenty-five years, had shrouded herself in excesses of indulgence, her husband developed a new admiration for her.

Conversation between the two became lively as Joyce explored her new feelings about the world around her. She began to introduce her husband to a part of the universe which he, for all his wordliness, had not known. For she introduced him to the pursuit of health and beauty, as well as knowledge.

LOOK YOUNGER - LOOK PRETTIER

In some marriages there are problems which are not based on personality differences so much as friction arising from an inability on the part of one or the other partner to relax. This lack of ease with oneself quickly carries over to the other, and actions of the affected person can become an irritant which in its own way can destroy a relationship.

Jean's problem was one of minor proportions, but of major consequences. Jean's husband felt driven from their bed on more than one occasion because his wife gritted her teeth at night in her sleep. His own irritation was manifested in a lack of sleep. Her insistence that he must be imagining that she had such a nerve-wracking habit, only irritated him further.

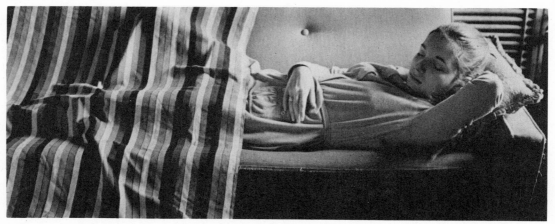

Jean's tenseness over daily living was bringing about the rending noises while she slept. No matter what decision she had to make during the course of a day, she panicked. She would check with her family and her friends before she would make a decision. This uncertainty and vacillation created suspense which she thought she disposed of. But in fact, she merely pushed it from her mind for the moment. At night while asleep, all of the unresolved attitudes and the indecisiveness of her nature swept forth. Her husband said sometimes her features were distorted from the intense frowning that accompanied the tooth-grinding.

When Jean turned to Yoga exercises and deep breathing, she found the relaxation and serenity that restored harmony to this marriage. Once she learned to concentrate, to keep her attention focused on one problem long enough to understand it, she found she could arrive at the best solution. This cannot take place if the mind remains uncontrolled, and flits restlessly about. Deep breathing, learning to slow down one's actions, and the sense of well-being that comes from regular physical exertion, all worked together here.

HOW YOGA SAVED THREE MARRIAGES

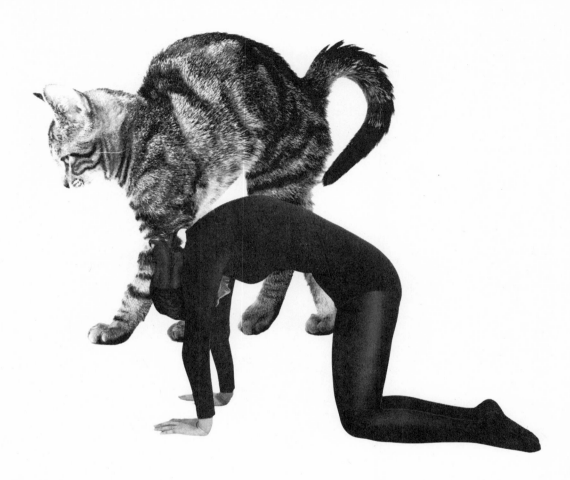

The Cat

Kneel on the hands and the knees so that the back is parallel to the floor and the palms of the hands are on the floor. Inhale and bring the head down to the chest, humping the back up like a cat. Suck up the stomach toward the spine and hold the breath as long as possible. Relax the body.

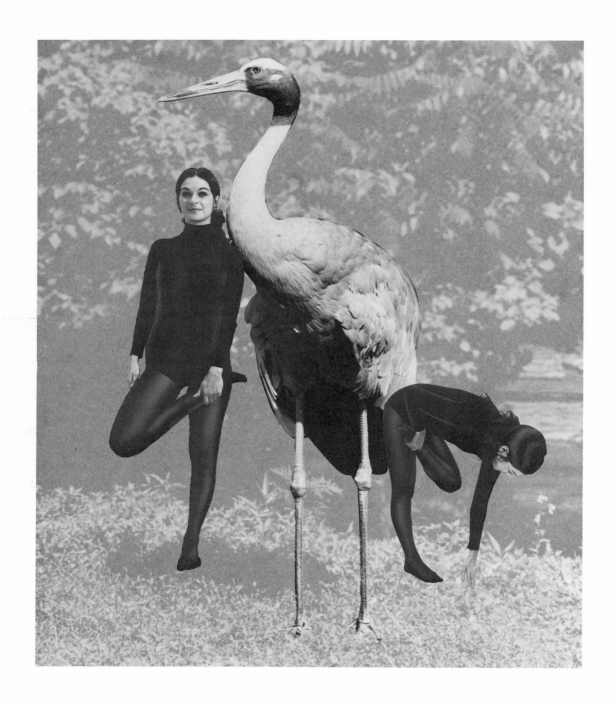

The Stork I *(far left)*

Stand upright and slowly raise the right leg and bend it at the knee. Hold the foot of the right leg with the left hand, keeping it in front of the thigh. Remain in this position while deep breathing in and out. Relax. Repeat with the left leg and the right hand, deep breathing all the while.

The Stork II *(left)*

Begin in the same upright position as in Step I. As you exhale, bend at the waist and bring the palm of the hand down to the floor. Hold this position as long as possible as you breathe in and out before returning to the standing position.

Repeat, using the opposite leg and hand.

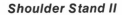

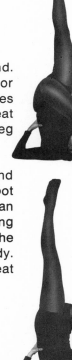

Shoulder Stand II

Step A

Go into the regular shoulder stand. Now drop one leg at a time to the floor behind the head. Exhale as the leg comes down. Inhale and bring the leg up. Repeat with the other leg. Practice with only one leg at a time.

Step B

Go into the regular shoulder stand and continue through Step A. With one foot behind the head and the other leg in an upright position, hands firmly supporting the back, slowly swing the foot that is on the floor around in a wide arc behind the body. Return to an upright position, and repeat with the other leg.

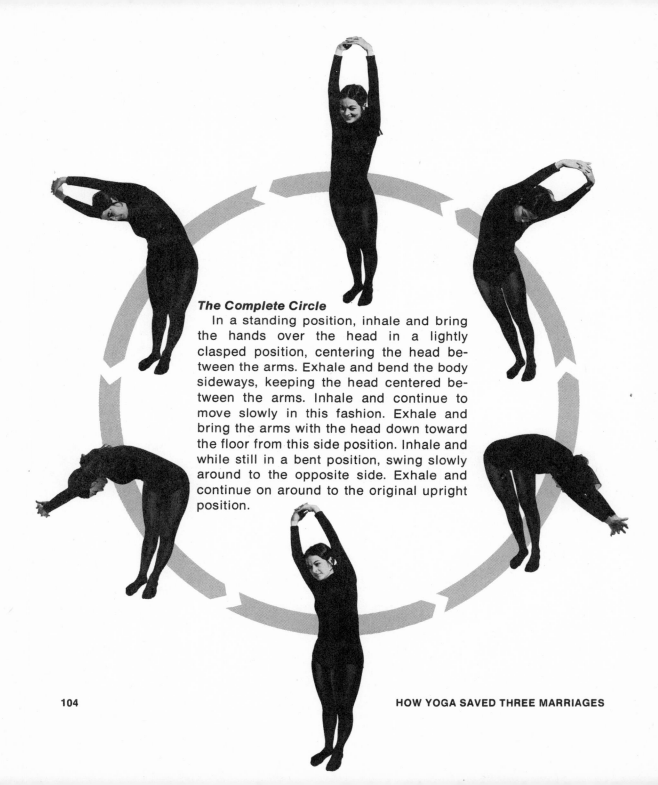

The Complete Circle

In a standing position, inhale and bring the hands over the head in a lightly clasped position, centering the head between the arms. Exhale and bend the body sideways, keeping the head centered between the arms. Inhale and continue to move slowly in this fashion. Exhale and bring the arms with the head down toward the floor from this side position. Inhale and while still in a bent position, swing slowly around to the opposite side. Exhale and continue on around to the original upright position.

EXERCISE BENEFITS IN CHAPTER 9

The Cat—The Cat tones the area of the arms and the back, plus the abdominal muscles. Toning of the sex organs is an additional benefit from the Cat. In addition, the movement is good for curing elimination problems.

The Stork—This two-part exercise brings about a balance that should be natural to the body. The alternate one-leg stance helps to establish equilibrium, which is further increased with the placing of the palm on the floor while guiding the body downward from a position on one leg.

Shoulder Stand II—This second part of the Shoulder Stand brings increased control of the body. Added mobility of the hips comes from the sweeping circular movement.

The Complete Circle—This complete and all-encompassing sideways movement carries the upper body in a full circle, for stimulation and a blood-flush to the face.

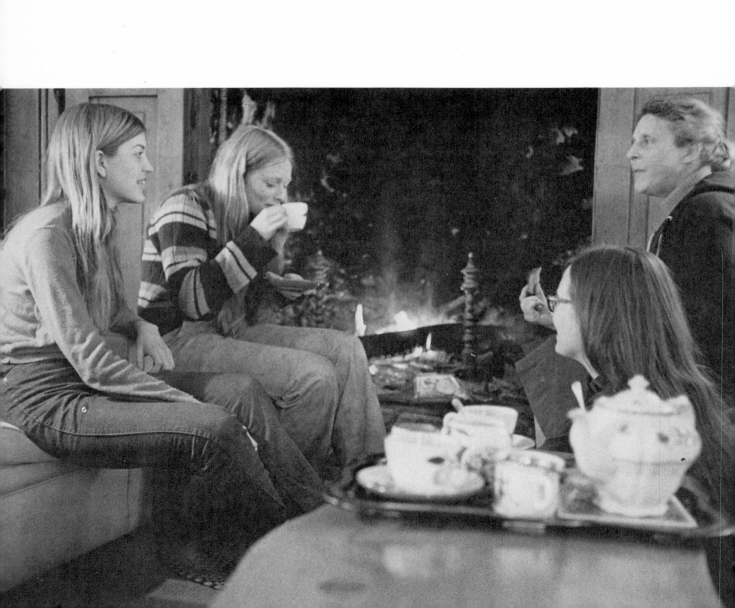

CHAPTER TEN - HOLD A YOGA KAFFEE KLATSCH!

How much of Yoga is acceptable to the average person? Is it possible to have a full and satisfying life without practicing the discipline of Yoga? The answer to these questions usually comes as a surprise.

Anyone who enjoys a good physical and mental poise is practicing a form of Yoga—whether he knows it or not—for it is not possible to remain in good health without adhering to the tenets of this practical discipline. The stalwart healthy man who says, "Yoga? Not on your life. No exotic Eastern culture for me!" is practicing Yoga, though he knows it by another name.

He walks the half mile to the commuter's station each morning and returns the same way every evening. He passes up the martinis and manhattans at lunch and chooses a vegetable soup, a crisp and refreshing salad and some form of fruit for dessert. Or better yet, he opens his briefcase at lunch to expose a nutritious home-prepared midday meal.

When he returns home he does not sink into the softest chair and turn on the television set, or hide behind the newspaper or a magazine. Instead, he clips his hedges, mows his lawn, rakes the leaves, or performs some other type of work that takes him away from the problems he faced at work all day.

If he is inclined towards sports, he is involved in some other outdoor project that holds his chest back and causes him to breathe deeply. In consequence, he sleeps peacefully at night and rises refreshed in the morning.

This is all a form of Yoga, for Yoga suggests that one tend to the body and care for it by working it rather than pampering it.

Another person who would be surprised to hear that she is practicing Yoga is the serene woman, delicate in her movements, who thinks that Yoga is practiced by scantily clad but heavily turbaned East Indians who, as caricatures suggest, spend their time climbing unsecured ropes.

But this same woman rises to an early morning swim or a brisk walk. After a simple and nourishing breakfast, she dresses for an active day that may include a full day's occupation at home, in an office, or in a shop. She will move her body naturally and easily, because she knows the value of a limber physique. She will avoid the chair that is too comfortable, preferring one with a straight back that offers a framework for her shoulders should she momentarily forget and sink back in a curved manner.

This woman, too, will avoid the cocktail for lunch, and will accept a vegetable juice instead. She will choose wisely from a menu created more for the lustful eye than the intelligent mind. Somewhere among all the creamed, mayonnaised and gravied foods, white breads, rolls, and sauced dishes, she will find one or two basic foods. Perhaps a hardboiled-egg salad with oil and vinegar dressing on it. Or a bowl of soup, or cheeses and fruits. But whatever she avoids, and whatever she chooses, she keeps in mind at all times that nutrition is a major part of good living. Knowing this, and accepting it, she will not try to cheat herself by imposing unnecessarily rich or useless foods on her body.

At no time will she close her eyes and her mind to her nutritional needs. The short-lived artificial pleasure she might know for a moment's deviation from the path of good health would not make up for the debt her body will have to pay for an unwise decision.

These people are practicing a form of Yoga. So is the person who props his feet on a desk in order to rest himself. Etiquette says: "Horrors!" Yoga says: "Excellent!" This method of restoring vigor to a fatigued body puts into effect the ancient Yogaic technique for reversing the gravity flow, and its subsequent pull on the body.

There is an economy of movement in Yoga exercises. No laboring, exhaustive propulsions of the body can be found in any asana. With an overall design of flexing every part of the human body, the movements of each and every Yoga exercise might be compared to the practical workings of a watch. Exactly what is needed is there, and nothing else.

Yoga is becoming a household word. From its early introduction in this country when a select few gathered to try this discipline so different from body-bending sports practices, it has grown to attract men and women all over the country. No longer the province of an exotic few, Yoga has become recognized as a rejuvenator, bringing clarity of thought and impetus to living even as it restores one's body to exhilarating health.

Yoga To Start A Day

In this busy, hurried life, kaffe klatsches have wide appeal. But such friendly gatherings snare a great many victims and encourage damaging eating habits that can destroy one's day. A group of women in one neighborhood would gather at one or another's house, according to convenience, as soon as the last kindergartner had been put on the bus and the last husband had darted for the local train.

They would come prepared to share a pot of coffee, to discuss those events that

HOLD A YOGA KAFFEE KLATSCH!

had transpired since the morning before, and to consume freshly baked coffee cake or even a commercial brand, thickly laced with confectioner's sugar or buttered crumbs. They felt this pleasant beginning would give them impetus to get on with the day's work.

With coffee, cake, and cigarettes, one to two hours could be whiled away in this style. Discussion ranged over a limited field of topics. According to one participant, their conversations covered anything that had occured in the last twenty-four hours within their own families. Margot said even she could hardly believe the quality of the conversation in which she took a part. It was idle chatter, meant to relax one. But it seldom accomplished this goal. By the time several cups of coffee had been consumed, sweetened with sugar, along with the tempting coffee cake spread with butter, there was, more likely, a case of coffee nerves that would play havoc with the remainder of the day.

These morning meetings were an escape, Margot suggested, from the humdrum reality of their secure and unexciting lives.

"We thought we were adding a sparkle to our days by meeting in each others' homes and gossiping about trivia," she recalls.

But as time went on, the sparkle that might have been there for some, lessened with repetition, and Margot and her friends discussed possible alternatives to their kaffee klatsches.

"We weren't really a group of idle-minded women, but rather a group of women without a sense of direction. We discussed forming a literary club, or commitments of another form. But many of the group already belonged to one or more charitable organizations or social groups, and felt they would not be interested in joining yet another. We liked each other's company, but our gathering together daily seemed to grow more meaningless, and yet, we had nothing with which to replace it.

"So we decided to look the problem squarely in the face. The problem was us. We came to the next morning kaffee klatsch as agreed, with pen and paper in hand. And we each chose one person at a time and started taking stock of her. It was a rough inventory, and we were all quite frank, as we had agreed to be."

The results spared no one.

Margot was listed as "heavy in the hips, beginning to develop a double chin, thick ankles, and smoking too much." Others in the group fared little better, for the inventory had to be honest in order to be effective. Even personalities were remarked on. Several of the women were labeled as quick-tempered. Others in the morning group were termed brusque, inconsiderate of others, boastful of their own and their children's accomplishments, or indifferent about their appearance.

Since these women hoped to benefit from the honest appraisal, there was no malicious intent in the stock-taking. This was their moment to help one another, and to be honest at the same time without losing a friendship. The individual papers were all gathered together and handed to each woman in turn. No one was expected to read the papers aloud if she chose not to. But they all submitted to this and felt that any attempt to discount the comments could be valid only if everyone present disagreed with them.

Most of the comments came as a rude shock. But there was no use being an ostrich about it. If they were genuinely concerned, then it was up to them to change this unflattering picture that they obviously presented, not only to their own group of morning coffee drinkers, but to the world at large and especially to their own families.

The next step obviously was some form of self-improvement approach. Many of the women had heard of Yoga, but thought of it mostly as an exotic meditative practice. But one of the women in the group had read a book on Hatha Yoga and its benefits and persuaded the others that this was what they needed. She convinced her friends that discipline was what they all needed, and that Yoga instilled this.

Arrangements were made to engage a Yoga teacher to come once a week to early morning kaffee klatsch to give an hour's instruction. For the remaining four days they met as usual. But instead of sitting around the table drinking coffee, smoking, and eating coffee cake, they practiced their week's exercises. They even gave up the usual refreshment, for some of those personal comments still rankled, and it is not as easy to swallow a sizable chunk of buttery cake when one knows someone in the group has said about you, "Heavy in the hips."

Bodies began to take on tone. Several women who had taken their measurements upon commencing, spoke of lost inches in the waistline within a couple of weeks. Without doubt there was constant improvement going on among them. Even those who had had no glaring figure faults, but had been noted for a shortness of temper, or a gloominess of attitude, began to note a change.

After two months, the group decided to stop meeting daily for their exercise practices. They decided to exercise individually at home and to meet just once a week instead, thus giving them more time to pursue new interests. The time that had been filled so casually before now took on a more important meaning. There was an enthusiasm among the women to enlarge their mental pursuits. This comes about when the body is put in good order and the mind is free to rise out of the everyday trivia of living. When the mind is released completely, with no clamor from an aching, overweight or tense body, then expansion of thought will come more easily. Time becomes available for accomplishments that would otherwise be impossible.

The kaffee klatsch group enjoyed their weekly meetings far better now. There were things of substance to share. There were courses to take to increase one's knowledge, reading to do for an expanded awareness, and areas where one could help another and gain the wonderful uplift that generosity always brings.

The practice of Yoga has long been recommended for creating poise in the awkward body. Once freed from stiffened joints and tautened ligaments, almost anyone can develop a beautiful carriage.

Diane was attracted to the stage as a young girl when she accompanied her mother to Saturday matinees. For years she had watched the re-creation of scenes representing real life enacted on the stage before her. And she had been drawn to the carefully enunciated speech and the deliberate movements of the body that the actors employed to interpret the emotions of a scene.

Diane would return home and repeat all of the lines from the play she could recall. Thus she began to prepare for her eventual entry into the domain of drama. The stage and its magic became her world, and it was here that she planned to place all of her interests. She worked hard in preparation for her career on the stage. Her speech was exquisite. Her many hours of practice before a mirror to an imagined audience had its rewards. Full-bodied and rich, her voice could command all the emotions that produce anger, fear, joy, or sorrow, with equal facility.

But her one area of weakness was an important one. Her body remained stiff and uncompromising, even with all her practiced striding across a stage. This eventually brought her to a Yoga class in an effort to loosen her movement and create a more pliable body.

When the script called for Diane to stride purposefully across a room, she appeared to stomp across. She could not seem to coordinate her movements enough to attain the ease required of her. When an easy gait was the stage direction, Diane was so awkward that she appeared to be rocking across the stage. As far as meaningful movements with the arms, she admitted she was quite capable of swinging out and striking someone inadvertently when she was attempting an expressive stage gesture.

Diane's problem was not a difficult one for Yoga to correct. Her awkwardness would disappear when she learned to control her body with daily exercises that would reduce her tenseness. She was impatient, however, for results, and had to be reminded of the many years she had moved her body in this awkward manner. Her stiffness could not be changed as rapidly as she would have liked. And she had to carry out daily practice of her positions in order to achieve the effortless walk that permitted her freedom to perform well on the stage.

Constantly reminding herself that without daily performance, no results could be expected, Diane eventually was rewarded. Application of all the Yoga exercises, including the Leg Stretch, which helps extend hamstrung muscles, created an easily-moving Diane. She learned to enter a room and turn, stop, glide, or saunter across it without mishap, or the sensation, as she described it, of being on somebody else's legs.

With an awkwardness of movement gone, Diane could concentrate on executing her roles in a manner that could conceivably take her where she wanted to go in the world of theater.

The discomfort of an aching back can stamp even the prettiest features with grimaces of pain. Curtailment of movement from this physical condition narrows one's life and affects adversely the manner in which one approaches each day.

Ann had suffered back pain since before her first child was born. Her years as a young mother and wife had been marred by this discomfort which seldom subsided and never disappeared. She learned to avoid any movement that might worsen these aches that were referred to as "low back pain."

On particularly bad days, Ann took aspirin or some narcotic pain-deadener. She actually came to prefer those days when she had to reach for the pain-killer pills. At least then her nerves were completely deadened to feeling, and she could begin to move about more easily.

But Ann knew that continued reliance on the drugs she was using would create new problems, and noting her growing dependency on them, she looked for ways of helping herself out of the discomfort of a weak back. Active sports as a means of strengthening her back could not be considered. Finally, the moderate movements of westernized Yoga, with its postures that she herself could control at all times, were suggested to her.

By the end of her first class, Ann could easily perform the breathing exercises. She informed the instructor of her back problem and she was cautioned to perform the exercises only once each day, for at least two weeks, and after that, dependent on her reaction, she could proceed as she chose.

She patiently watched as other students repeated the same exercise. She resisted the impulse to perform them more than the one suggested time, although they were pleasantly stimulating. Gradually she worked up to repeating the exercises without adverse effects, and her sense of well-being increased with practice.

The exercise she preferred and felt brought her the greatest reward was that of the Twist. This all-encompassing movement almost turned her into a human pretzel, with many beneficial movements to the body that she had not experienced before. Pitting one muscle against another, the Twist is one of the oldest forms of isometric exercise, since in point of origin it dates back two or more centuries.

It was in this slow and orderly fashion that Ann overcame the low back pain that had plagued her for years. There were other benefits, too. Enough of them for Ann finally to arouse her husband's enthusiasm and that of her children. With the entire family practicing Yoga, they have safeguarded their health; instead of waiting for an ailment or discomfort to commence, they ward it off by the good health practices of Yoga.

Head Stand I

Kneel and place the head on the floor, specifically the area which is just above the forehead. This would be the centered area between the middle of the head and the middle of the forehead. Clasp the hands with fingers interlocking and place them behind the head. They will form a kind of cup for the back of the head. Keep the hands and the forearms on the floor. The elbows must lie immediately beside the knees. Do not allow your head to rest *in* your hands, but rather *against* your hands. As you go up into your position, your hands must not be *under* your head; that would be incorrect. They must be *behind* the head, serving as a barrier of sorts.

Take one small step back and rise up on the toes, knees off the ground. The weight must be on the arms and the elbows, rather than on the head. Check this position and correct if necessary by beginning over. This is the first of three steps which will ultimately lead to the complete Head Stand. The two following steps will be presented in later lessons. This position is to be practiced daily for a minimum of a week. You may relax after the first effort, and repeat as many times as you like.

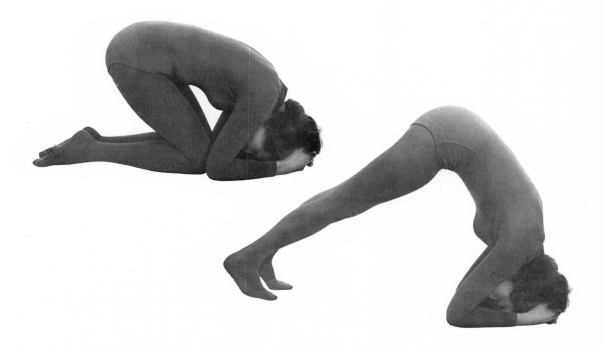

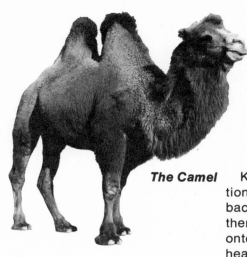

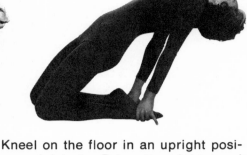

The Camel   Kneel on the floor in an upright position and inhale. Bring the right hand back onto the instep of the right foot, then bring the other hand backward onto the instep of the left foot. Allow the head to go backward as far as is comfortable. Deep breathe in and out while in this position. Then exhale and bring one hand up at a time as you resume a normal position.

Supine Pose (right)

Kneel on the floor, feet apart, and sit between your legs. Lean backward first on one elbow and then on the other, until full support is felt on both elbows. Roll the head backward until the top of the head rests off the floor. Keep the hands in the middle of the chest, palm against palm. Deep breathe going down, and inhale going up.

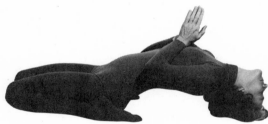

The Body Stretch

Standing with the legs apart, deep breathe and bring the arms over the head. Stretch and exhale and then bring the palms of the hands to the floor, or as close as possible to the floor. Tuck the head close to the knees.

If this pose is easily attained, then bring the feet closer together and proceed with the movement.

HOLD A YOGA KAFFEE KLATSCH!

EXERCISE BENEFITS IN CHAPTER 10

Headstand I—In this first approach to the full headstand, the correct placement of supportive hands and the position of the head, plus the proper weight distribution is practiced. A sense of balance is developed as one adjusts one's weight placement. Neck muscles are brought into play as the correct position is sought.

The Camel—In its reverse position, or opposite to the front bending movements, the Camel offers stimulation to the thyroid gland as the head is tilted backward. The vertebrae gain suppleness by this flexing position.

Modified Supine Pose—An expansion of the chest and a strengthening of the shoulders result from this unusual backward rolling of the head and the shoulders.

Body Stretch—The entire body receives a refreshing stretch in this tension-removing exercise. Suppleness of waist movement is increased and the spine is limbered. In addition, the muscles along the length of the leg receive fresh tone.

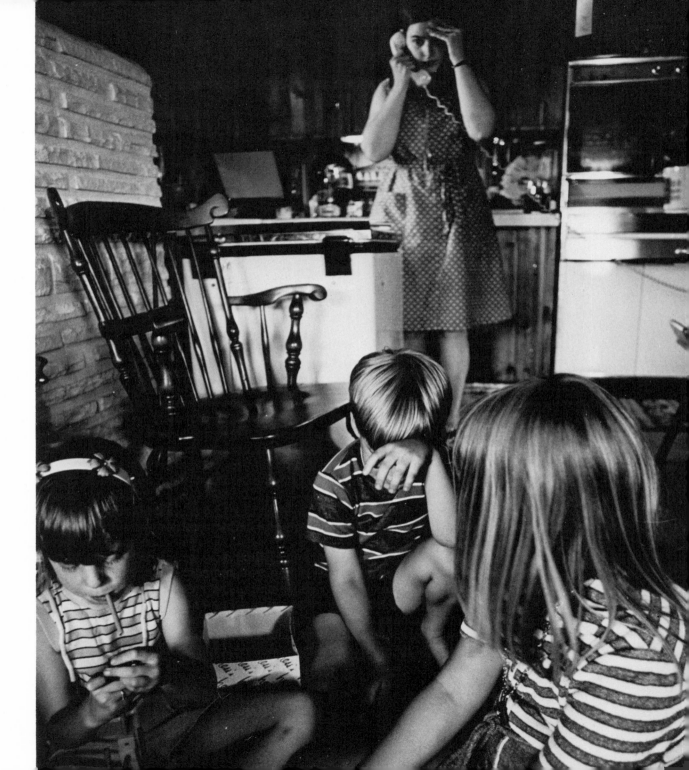

CHAPTER ELEVEN - CLOSING THE GENERATION GAP

Remembering Dr. Hans Selye's warning that civilized stress is a mass killer, it is easy enough to see also that strains imposed by today's changing cultures, if not adequately controlled, can destroy physical beauty. For natural beauty cannot be nurtured in an atmosphere that breeds tension and dissension.

There is no going backward in time, no hiding from the very real problems and issues of today. Parents with children in the home are going to be exposed more and more to new ideas, experiments in living, and changing values. This calls for adjustments, acceptance of new customs, and in general, a willingness to grow while holding on to values that have proved worthwhile.

Our country has grown increasingly tense, our people more uncertain of their aims and goals, and our state of health is dropping alarmingly.

Walk along any street in any small town or large city and search visually for a healthy-appearing person. What shall you search for? Look for slender bodies, without excess flesh or bulges at the waistline or abdomen, shoulder, chin, or cheek. Watch for good, clear skin, pleasant countenances, and apparent good humor, or a receptive or serene expression.

What do you find instead?

Almost without exception, overweight bodies, muddy complexions, and grim, bored, or hostile expressions.

And this is our world, the most affluent country of all—yet one that is growing increasingly unhealthy with the tensions of the time. The strain of daily living is taking its toll in lost working hours, broken homes, and a soaring criminal rate. Just as bad, inability to cope with strain makes the home a launch-pad for embittered personalities.

The distance between a younger and an older generation can sometimes become a gap over which few are prepared to leap. In short, many homes have become battlegrounds for the proving of strength. It is this futile battling, this conflict of personalities and clashing of wills that can bring about disasters more terrible than deprivation and physical want. The angers that are bred in such a household are destroyers of the mental calm that helps to create physical beauty. There is no use looking for health and beauty in a strictly physical sense. The two must work together hand-in-hand with *mental* health and beauty. The mind lays the groundwork for the external display of calm that removes lines from foreheads, releases tautly-held lips and lifts the shoulders upward.

If bitterness and despair cloud the eyes, no amount of make-up can conceal the grimly-held chin and the frowning face that ages more quickly than numerical years would dictate. Beauty must begin from within. In addition to the good nutrition and exercise that can cause a blossoming of beauty, there must be a willingness to adapt to today's exciting times. And here again, it is the mind that must lead the way. Without mental composure, complete deterioration of the body can follow from situations that spell despair for the unprepared.

The practice of Yoga can remove the fears that usually accompany change. Because of Yoga's harmonizing influence on the mind, no parent today should enter the arena of child-rearing and especially the challenge of teen-age years, without having practiced this discipline. In this fashion, not only will the muscular relaxation of Hatha Yoga increase the efficiency of living, with an economy of effort, but the calming influence of its practice will conserve and heighten the beauty that should belong to a woman in these years.

Pat's household was the scene of constant quarrelling, bitter resentments, and frustrations for every member of the family. At 38, Pat resembled a woman at least ten years older. And yet, her friends remembered her as a perenially youthful woman with incredible drive and a zest for each day's events. That was the picture that Pat had presented until two years ago.

Within that time, Pat had gone from the joyous, smoothly functioning woman voted "most likely not to have to worry about succeeding" in her senior year book, to the present aging and harried wife and mother.

Pat's formerly peaceful home continued to be the attractive residence she and her husband had built with thoughts of a family in mind. But in this carefully-planned setting, their two teenagers had become such an ordeal to Pat that she felt she might not even survive their complete upbringing.

Part of Pat's bitterness stemmed from the fact that until fairly recently - about two years ago - both youngsters had been the nucleus around which she revolved. She had reared her youngsters carefully and given them every opportunity to grow and expand, with herself always there to guide them in their decisions. They made no move without her watchful eye upon them, as she led them to better marks in school and an awareness of their duties as her children.

Pat felt some sort of dry rot had entered her Eden when the youngsters first began to rebel, to question her pronouncements regarding their lives. She quickly tried to sweep away the resistance, and to keep them on the path that was best for them, the path that they themselves would choose if their thinking had been more mature.

She did not understand the persistence of her daughter and son in adopting attitudes so different from hers. How could they possibly be attracted to the strange mores and codes of their schoolmates? Why did they want to take part in the general disobediences of the day? This would not advance their future. Therefore, she felt she must prevent them from making mistakes in their younger years.

Pat organized herself and planned full schedules designed to straighten the youngsters out and present them with true values. But somehow, the stronger her presentation, the more labor and planning that went into her organized strategies to turn them away from the dissident faction in their school, the more the youngsters seemed attracted to just those people. And the more adamant they became in pursuit of "causes."

Soon Pat was lying awake nights waiting for the sound of their return. Or if she heard a siren during the night she would find herself stumbling toward their rooms hoping to find them in bed, but all the while knowing they were both out on their separate missions.

Pat decided the time had come for increased firmness. She had always been in charge of the children, having shown her husband that this role was more suited to her than to him, with his busy life. In fact, she had encouraged him to be more a friend to the children than anything else, for what need had they for discipline?

Now Pat tried to slip from her role of gentle guide to a new role of stern dictator. She insisted and she informed. This was the way they were to behave in the future. There would be no more rebellion as to her decisions on hours to be home, or activities and acquaintances to be avoided.

However, Pat did not succeed in gaining control of her household with this more severe attitude. Instead, she was met with increased rebellion and indifference to her ultimatums. Eventually, her resentment came to rival that of her children. Her formerly pleasant voice became shrill. She began to scream. The household became the scene of daily verbal battles.

When one of her friends finally persuaded Pat that the open hostility from her children was more than a nerve-shattered woman could handle, Pat agreed to try to learn to calm herself by practicing Yoga.

In turning back to herself, Pat was able to give up some of the domineering clutching at her youngsters. She became involved in learning to breath deeply in order to avoid a mounting rage in their presence. As she ceased screaming in a shrill voice, life in her household calmed down.

Each time Pat noted defiance in one of her children, she learned to take deep breaths to calm herself. She also discovered by herself that the ordeal of confrontation with her children was not and could not be a solution. When they spoke of political attitudes opposite to hers, at first she relied on the deep breathing to avoid a hasty answer. After a while, when perfectly calm, she would ask for an explanation as to her child's preference or belief in his or her radical attitude.

When she asked, they told her. She said it was like taking bitter medicine at first, to hear them throw over all the values which she had tried to instill in them. But she was practicing tenets of Yoga that said she must listen to another's belief, even if that conviction was not her own. The simple rule she had taught her children years ago, "Do unto others," she was now learning to apply to herself.

Her own growth came with learning to listen quietly, even respectfully, not so much to their beliefs, as to their rights to voice them. Life in her home did eventually return to some of its former harmony. But there was a difference. Pat had been the dominant personality in her home before. Now the emerging personalities of her children took the lead, as though bursting out from under a nurturing pot that had held them as seedlings without permitting them to develop.

Pat never subscribed to her children's ideas of how to run the world, what personal freedom should include, nor, indeed, very many of their ideas at all. But she learned to respect her children's right to explore, to learn, and to seek unhampered mental growth without having her stamp of approval. She learned to listen without condemning. Because she became a calmer person, and no longer shouted in frustration at her children, their own defiance slackened. There was a growing sense of maturity in both mother and children.

Unable to communicate with her children once their minds began to develop more fully, Pat now learned that her own relaxed body and composed mind could open the way to, if not mental rapport, then at least, mental contact with the children she loved. And with her continued practice of Yoga, Pat gained the admiration of her children, because they saw an Establishment person willing to join their search for a better world, even though hers was projected from a different angle.

Rosalind's problem also stemmed from the changing times.

Finding herself alone without any demands other than those she placed on herself, Rosalind attempted to live her latter years of widowhood as she had lived the previous years that had been rich and full with concerns of rearing a family and being companion to her husband. The days that had never seemed long enough to accomplish what she had in mind, now lengthened intolerably.

With no requests from anyone, and without a sense of direction, Rosalind fast was becoming a person whose interests were turned inward. She dwelled upon her loneli-

CLOSING THE GENERATION GAP

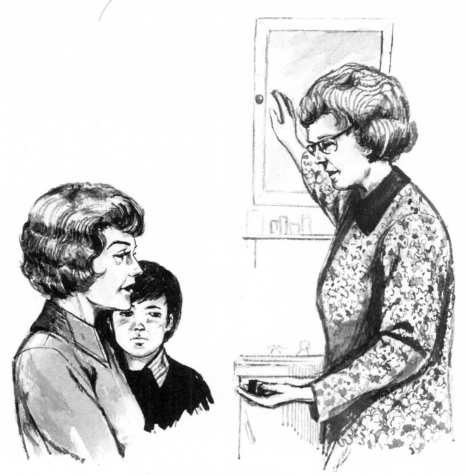

Pat and Rosalind

ness, her feeling of inadequacy, of no longer being needed by her family. She became conscious of any deviation in her physical feelings, and catered to her slightest indisposition.

In her vacuum, Rosalind began to turn more and more to herself as a source of need. Her medicine cabinet became well stocked with bottles aimed at reducing tension, nervousness, and exhaustion. In her occasional conversations with others, she began to direct the conversations toward herself, and her various illnesses.

By the end of her first year of being alone, Rosalind noticed that she was asked less and less often to join others in social gatherings. Bitterly attributing this to her recent widowhood, she withdrew into what she thought was a state of self-sufficiency. But it was a lonely state, and she began to lose the charm that had attracted people to her through the past years.

People, she thought, were no longer gracious, kind or loving. They were self-centered, indifferent, and not content to live in a peaceful world. They were, rather, determined to create and bring chaos to an established living order.

Persuaded by her children to add something of interest to her days, she read some literature on Yoga they brought her. Though the subject matter appeared rather exotic to her, she wanted the fulfillment of which Yoga spoke. She wanted also to be able to return to the feeling of completeness that she had known in earlier times. She continued to read various books on Yoga and to practice the simple but positive attitudes about which she read.

Then she learned of a course on Yoga and joined the group. She was surprised to find that the class was composed of teenagers, as well as of men and women in their forties, fifties, and sixties. It was here that Rosalind learned to meet today, and to relinquish her hold on yesterday.

Though she didn't grow overnight, there were discussions that she found stimulating, and in which she joined. She learned to listen to the young voices as well as the older ones. For people searching for a way of life, Rosalind learned that there could be no condemnation of another because of a difference in thinking, or a difference in years. She learned that the path that would lead to fulfillment and reason for living could be stepped upon at any point, by anyone who was searching.

As her physical health grew better, Rosalind's mental outlook was refreshed and improved. Her body developed more youthful lines, and she lost her various aches and pains; her mind became more alert and receptive to change.

Today Rosalind is busy with life. She is involved with people and is enjoyed for her attractive appearance no less than for her youthful ideas. She is busy doing things for people, rather than waiting for someone to notice her in her solitude.

Rosalind has gone to the world instead of waiting for the world to come to her.

Not everyone who decides to practice Yoga has a distinct or even a slight problem. Some turn to this age-old way of life as a means of enhancing their own life; of adding an unknown factor that may well expand their self-satisfaction. Others simply act from a subconscious desire to know life more fully; to be ready to acknowledge a way of life that may differ from the quiet routine of one's earlier years. In other words, some turn to the practice of Yoga from a sense of healthy curiosity about what else life might offer one if one seeks.

Marie had reached the age of fifty when she began to question the meaning of her past years.

"Life was so easy for me. It always has been. Someone has taken care of me since my earliest days. As a child, there were my parents. Then my husband was there to guide and decide, or help me to decide. After he passed away, my sons and daughters stepped in and advised me and helped me to continue living as I always had lived: uncommitted to any real involvement with life, and unaware of any emotion other than what was personal."

Marie was not unhappy during those years when someone was doing most of her thinking for her. Life was serene and without turmoil. But then, she decided, the life of a vegetable is also serene.

And while peace and serenity are something greatly to be desired, they are not to be accepted if they exclude purposeful living. We must acknowledge a need to transcend life's trivia and advance spiritually in a personal way.

Marie's cloistered existence shut her away from any depth of living, and eliminated all satisfaction of accomplishment. It was with a sense of shock that she acknowledged that she had never experienced anything that made her grateful to be alive.

"Satisfied, yes. But grateful for life itself, no."

Marie began to question her way of life, and her answers had to come from something other than the usual novels and popular magazines of the day that she consumed. Marie was seeking for depth, and for a reason to continue living. For each day had become tiresome to her now that duty was no longer there to occupy her mind. No one needed her, and she seemed to need no one. Within such a vacuum, life became meaningless.

Marie turned to various social activities and quickly tired of them before she finally found Yoga as a discipline that would commit her to life. One doesn't have to renounce his ways, or suddenly stop or start doing something, or nothing. One comes into Yoga so easily, she found.

Yoga awakened Marie from her lethargical, meaningless days. Now she uses her mind as more than a sponge for soporific reading matter. She is alive as never before, and she has become aware of her body and her mind. She remains comfortable and serene. But with a new dimension added to her life; she is involved with people and her awakened curiosity has endowed her with a genuine affinity for living.

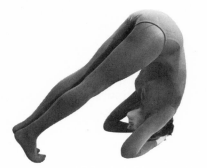

Headstand II

Review Headstand I and check to determine if the weight is on the arms and elbows.

In Step II, walk one step forward and straighten the legs. This creates a change in weight, so be sure the weight is kept on the arms and elbows. The torso will now be in a virtually perpendicular position.

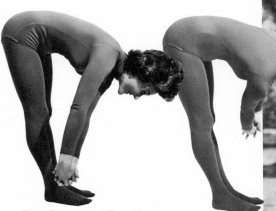

The Elephant Trunk

While in a standing position, inhale and bring both arms over the head. Exhale and bend down from the waist. Allow the hands to swing back and forth from the heel of one foot to the heel of the other foot, without touching the floor. This will create a semi-circular movement that moves both the shoulders and the arms in a slightly twisting position. Breathe in and out, and on exhalation, return to a standing position.

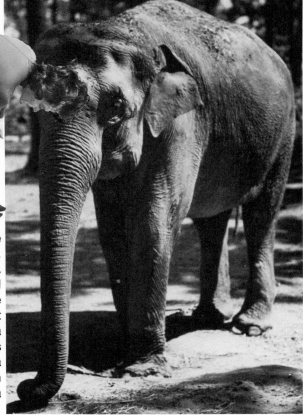

124

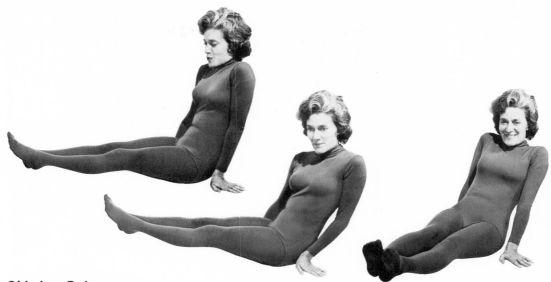

Side Leg Raise

Sit on the floor with the legs directly out in front with your hands at your sides. Lift both legs off the floor about six inches. Deep breathing in and out, move the legs from the right to the left. Keep an even distance from the floor during the entire movement. Return the legs to the floor on an exhaled breath.

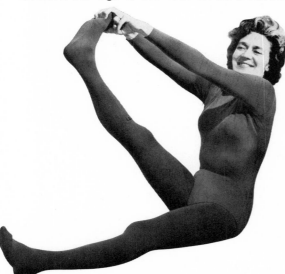

Leg Stretch

Sit on the floor with both legs held straight before you. Bend one knee, and hook the index and third fingers around the big toe. Bring the foot up in the air until the knee is straight. Do not slant the body. Inhale while lifting the leg upward, and exhale when bringing it down. Repeat the same with the other knee.

LOOK YOUNGER - LOOK PRETTIER

EXERCISE BENEFITS IN CHAPTER 11

Headstand II—This is a continued preparation for the full Headstand which teaches a changing of weight distribution to insure proper balance in the final posture. Its benefits, as we shall later see, are many.

Elephant Trunk—This asana eliminates body tension by the easy swinging movements of the arms, waist and shoulders.

Side Leg Raise—A disciplined balance of the body which requires the lifting of the legs a few inches off the floor while in a seated position. Leg and back muscles are stimulated, and the hip area receives increased agility by this performance.

Leg Raise—Muscles from the thigh down to the toes are employed in this movement. Back muscles and ligaments are toned with this exercise that also aids in relieving hamstrung muscles in the leg.

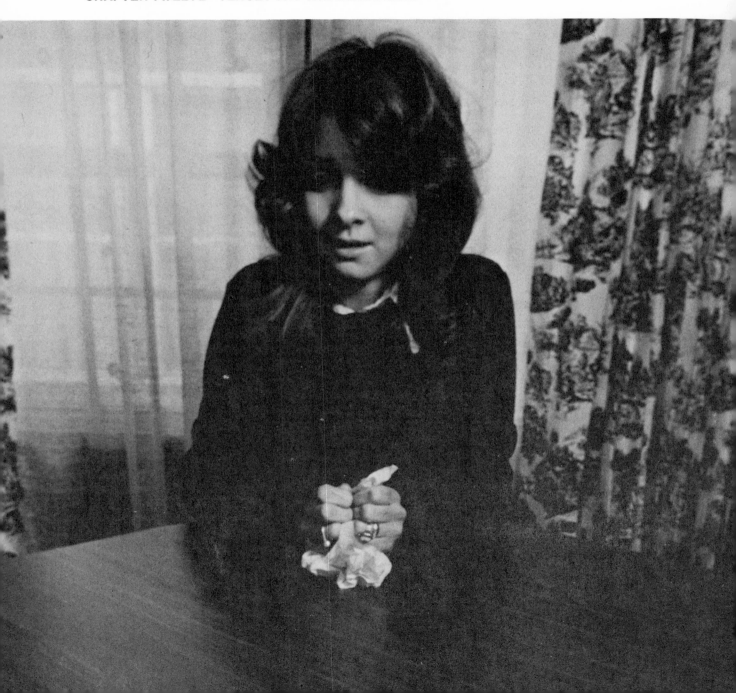

Persons who have a concern about health fall into one of two categories: those intent upon gaining health, and those interested in maintaining health. And yet the rules for these two groups are one and the same. One cannot stage a permanent return to health after an illness without utilizing the same practices that sustain and guard good health in the first place.

Yoga practices, sensibly followed, can restore the vibrancy of life, and if the same rules that brought about the rescue of the body are faithfully adhered to after the return

So little is required of this discipline that gives so much. Anyone who follows the rules of Yoga cannot fail to benefit from them. With faithful practice of the various exercises, and new awareness of oneself and the natural laws that govern the body, improved health and beauty are sure to follow.

In our society today we look for nostrums and quick remedies that will not make us use our bodies. This in itself is shortsightedness, for by failing to use the body properly, one extends an open invitation to premature aging, illness, and mental deterioration. And the less the body is put to use, the more it rebels when demands are placed upon it; until finally, muscles and ligaments sink more and more into a state of torpor, taking from the mind the keen edge of awareness.

Our bodies are our most important possession. And yet, do we not pay more attention and give more care to other possessions? We paint our homes, mow our lawns, feed and nourish our plants, and keep a careful check on appliances to be certain that we get as much use as possible out of them.

For our bodies, we take a quick shower, grab a bite to eat, take a brief nap, jump into the car, race to the store, and rush home.

If one will pause along this disastrous route to assess himself and the fate to which he is pushing his body, the need for remedial action will become apparent. No matter how damaged the body, no matter how betrayed by ill living and neglect, there is some aspect that can be reclaimed and bettered. We are not speaking of irreversible physical handicaps, though some of these, too, can be eased by simple, easy exercises. We are emphasizing rather the need to halt the toll that a neglected and abused body must pay, for lack of intelligent use.

Merely by learning to deep breathe, one can avoid some diseases of the respiratory tract. Wastes that accumulate from shallow breathing can be expelled by the more cleansing, deeper breaths.

Those with heart difficulties find that the moderate movements of Yoga will help to improve their health in ways forbidden calisthenics never could. Older persons who have reached a point of ill health that permits little or no locomotion can still benefit from postures that require a minimum of body movement. The Lion, deep breathing, eye exercises, and hand postures are some of the many helpful movements that bring increased agility to the body that is reduced to sub-normal activity.

Other exercises offer a gentle massaging action to the inner organs. In this manner, better digestion can take place in the stomach. This same massaging can stimulate the intestines and relieve gaseous distresses from poorly digested food. Even the most nourishing foods require a sound digestive system if they are to be fully utilized by the body.

For those suffering from sinus congestion, hay fever, or asthma, the need for an opened nasal area sometimes becomes so great that at times one would pay the greatest price asked just to be able to breathe again without obstruction.

Of inestimable value in such distresses, the headstand offers stimulation to those areas that by the natural laws of gravity would be receiving a diminished blood supply when in an upright position.

The Headstand can and does clear up many respiratory distresses. My own seasons of raging rose fever, commencing each spring and lasting through the summer months, were cured by practicing the headstand daily. So bad was my rose fever that during those months of drifting pollen, my movements outdoors were greatly curtailed. I became chained to a box of Kleenex.

Though I had suffered from rose fever for a number of years, it reached its peak while my husband and I were living in St-Cloud, just outside Paris. Beyond my terrace, there was a magnificent tree. Each spring the tree let loose a myriad of feathery spirals which drifted wing-like around the entire neighborhood. Because one seldom if ever finds window screens in France, and never in Paris, the pollen on the feathery mass flew through opened windows and covered the floors. One could keep his window and doors closed, but this shut out the lovely breezes and charming sounds. On occasion I had to stand near the tree, waiting for the bus. I had to wet several handkerchiefs and hold them over my nostrils in order to avoid most of the irritating pollen.

The condition continued until I began to practice the Headstand. In a matter of weeks my allergy disappeared, and has never returned in the intervening years. The need to walk down the street with the familiar Kleenex box under one arm has long since disappeared.

The clearing up of allergies is not the only thing for which the Headstand must be praised. Complete release from tension will be noticed by many within minutes of going into this position. It is as though all exterior irritations cease when the inverted position is taken; but of course, they are still there. It is simply that one has, by this position, increased the flow of blood to areas of the body that might previously have received a meager supply. With the strengthened blood flow through the body, and specifically through neglected areas, there is a calming influence that relaxes both mind and body.

In consequence, tension seems to slip away. Upon assuming a normal position, one is much better equipped to handle one's problems than before. With a more alert mind, one can dispose of irritations before they become major problems. Therefore, it is wise to ward off the many assaults on the mind during the course of a day by taking a Headstand break at any time when pressures seem to be building around you.

Many people have found that a few minutes taken out in mid-morning or mid-afternoon to go into the Headstand will do far more to keep them alert and functioning than does the more usual coffee-break. Quickened mental activity is the reward if this position is practiced during a time of fatigue. The soothing flow of blood brings with it food for the mind that can never come from coffee or other artificial stimulants.

Many businessmen and women credit the Headstand with being one of their major sources of extra energy. With an increase in circulation, there is no doubt that one can profit from this vitality-producing asana.

For beauty purposes, the Headstand becomes invaluable. It would be to the owner's advantage if every beauty parlor in the country would institute a course in Yoga, with the Headstand the main attraction for one interested in the pursuit of beauty. All movements of Yoga lead to beauty, certainly, and the Headstand is high on the list.

Tributes paid to this posture are legion. And most of them, if indeed, not all, are merited. This rejuvenator of the mind also reverses the flow of gravity that pulls the tissues of the face downward all the hours of the waking day. Wrinkles are in part attributed to this constant pull on the face and the neck.

In order to lessen the effects of constant sagging due to gravity pull, daily practice of the Headstand serves admirably.

The list of benefits is long. The roots of the hair receive a beneficial treatment in this daily position. Since this is the last part of the body to receive nutrition, it quite obviously will produce a more luxuriant growth when there is increased circulation.

There are many other Yoga exercises that bring about improved health conditions. Positions that develop strength in the body and greater ease of movement of the limbs can help to eliminate discomforts of long standing.

Pains in her shoulders had sent Amy racing to her doctor. Amy operated a machine press where she worked to support her invalid husband and four children. With the oldest child in his senior year at school, Amy had felt on the threshold of something wonderful. No one in either her family or her husband's had ever had the opportunity for a higher education.

Amy was eager for her children to prepare well for the lives ahead of them. Because of the struggle they had always known, they held long discussions about their future. Each child had agreed to help the one younger than he. So all Amy had to do was to get her oldest son into college and assist him as she could. Then he would proceed to help the

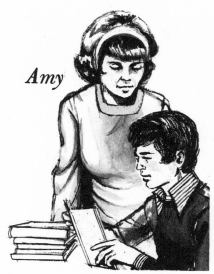

Amy

next in age when the time came for his college entrance. They would work for scholarships and find part-time jobs to enable them to meet their expenses.

Each child would help to lift up the one behind him, as he himself gained a more secure footing. Amy knew they would manage because they were accustomed to responsibility. But in order to put their plan into operation, Amy had to be able to contribute toward the overall expenses at least during the first years the older ones were at college. This would be in addition to supporting the younger ones still at home.

Amy, however, had another problem. The doctor diagnosed bursitis in her shoulders. This inflammation limited her movements of this part of the body. There was little relief for her in the weeks that followed. The inflammation would subside, only to flare up again without apparent reason.

Amy needed her job, but the constant shoulder movement involved in operating her equipment caused great suffering. Her son suggested Yoga as a means of learning to use the body correctly. He had taken a course at the local Y and practiced it at home. He spoke to his mother of the value of using the body in an overall manner, of giving it overall movement to compensate for the constant use of the shoulder area.

Amy replied that this seemed to be precisely the problem. She had overused one part of her body. Her son agreed with her.

Despite her busy life, Amy found the time necessary to begin daily practicing of Yoga postures. She was impatient with the movements at first, and could not perform any asanas which required full use of her shoulders. But Amy did not want her son to think she was a quitter. She practiced at home fifteen minutes before retiring each evening. Bit by bit the pain in her shoulders subsided during the following weeks. By the time two months had elapsed, Amy could lift her arms over her head—a feat that had been impossible since the pain had commenced.

She felt a moment of triumph when she managed to do the Cowhead Pose. For this required complete ease of movement of the shoulders. Amy could feel muscles called into play for the first time, and knew that the strength of her body would increase according to its movements.

Though now she still occasionally feels minor discomfort in the formerly inflamed area, Amy is able, with her continued practice of Yoga, to pursue her admirable plans for her family.

LOOK YOUNGER - LOOK PRETTIER

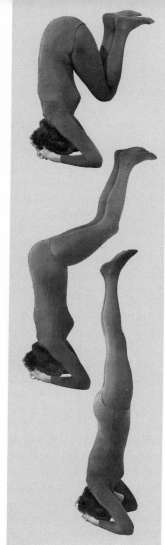

Full Headstand

Review Headstand I and II.

In Step III, bring the knees in to the chest. Allow the feet to leave the floor, as they fold with the soles upward. Knees pressed close to the chest, steady yourself in this half-headstand. This is the step in which you must strive for complete balance of your body.

Many students will not be able to accomplish this step the first time. Do not become discouraged. If there is hesitancy, or fear of falling, then the wisest place to practice is against the wall. In this instance, place your hands in their clasped position around the head about six inches from the wall. Go through Steps I and II. Now kick one leg upward toward the wall. This reassurance will enable you to bring up the other foot and gain the position of the headstand without fear of falling. After a few moments, slowly come down from the position.

To come down from the Headstand against the wall, place the soles of the feet flat against the wall and walk down until the knees are bent. Then let one foot leave the wall as the body bends at the waist. This slow movement will bring the body down easily.

To come down from the Headstand without benefit of the wall for support, simply fold the knees in toward the chest until the feet are aimed at the floor.

It is wise to remain in a prone position after coming down from the Headstand for the same length of time you were in the inverted positon. This is a vital part of the overall care that must be taken in performing the Headstand, and must be considered as part of the position itself in order to avoid any lightheadedness.

Inclined Plane (right)

Sit on the floor with your legs straight out in front of you. Place the arms straight behind you a few inches from the buttocks with the palms flat on the floor. Inhale and lift the buttocks off the floor. Arch the spine backward and roll the head backward. Feet must remain flat on the floor. Deep breathe in and out and return to a normal position on an exhaled breath.

Frog Pose

Take a position of kneeling, sitting between the legs. Spread the knees wide apart until the toes meet in back. Place the hands on the knees. Buttocks will be resting on the floor. Deep breathe in and out and remain in this position as long as it is comfortable, up to a full minute.

Cowhead Pose

Take a position of kneeling while sitting between the legs. Bring the right arm over the right shoulder. Extend the right hand down, between the shoulder blades, to reach the hand of the left arm which is also in back, bent at the elbow, and is reaching upward toward the right shoulder, left palm outward. Let the right hand reach for the left hand until the fingers interlock. Hold this position while deep breathing, relax, and repeat with the left arm reaching over the left shoulder and the right arm reaching up toward the left shoulder to meet the fingers of the left hand.

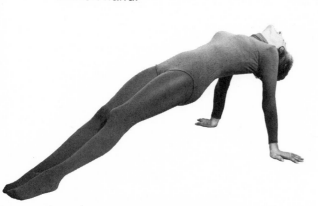

LOOK YOUNGER - LOOK PRETTIER

EXERCISE BENEFITS IN CHAPTER 12

Full Headstand—Offering benefits of the most comprehensive degree, the Headstand refreshes a fatigued body and mind. Circulation is improved by this inverted position; mental alertness returns to a dulled mind, and the mental powers are increased. Serenity flows from the development of self-confidence brought about by the Headstand. Nervous tension is diminished in this position, and an exhilaration of both body and mind takes place. In addition, the shoulders and arms are greatly strengthened, along with neck muscles. The downward pull on the abdominal area is reversed with the Headstand and this position provides a good treatment for a sagging abdomen.

Inclined Plane—This backward bending movement is an excellent abdomen stretch that also strengthens the back, shoulders, legs and arms.

Frog Pose—The thighs and calves are benefited in this leg-stretching exercise. Greater agility is obtained as the hips are flexed into position. Increased ease of movement is gained in walking, through the gradual stretching of the ankles.

Cowhead Pose—This posture offers firmness to the chest as the pectoral muscles are strengthened. Many find it useful for firming the breasts. In addition, the shoulders can be relieved of bursitis, or any condition of stiffness.

CHAPTER THIRTEEN - EXERCISES FOR SPECIFIC AREAS

Just as the whole body will benefit from strengthening exercises, the eyes, too, will profit from stimulation....if it is gentle. One frequently hears of a diagnosis of "lazy eye" from an optometrist. Usually a corrective or stronger lens is prescribed for the weakened orb. When one asks what has made the eye lazy, the answer most often given is that the organ is functionally weak, and that therefore, the affected person has shifted the search for vision to the stronger eye, furthering the neglect that helped create the problem.

Some optometrists recommend exercises. Many do not. But if the muscles of the eyes are weak, and this is the main cause of diminished eyesight, then one should spend a few minutes a day on the following method of restoring tone to the eye muscles, and in this manner help eliminate eye strain resulting from underexercised muscles.

Eye Exercises

Sit in an easy pose on the floor. Hold the spine erect while relaxing the body. Place the hands loosely across the thighs. Visualize the face of a clock so large that the numerals are out of sight of your eyes. In order to "see" the printed numerals, you will have to gaze as high and wide and low as you can, for in this practice, it is necessary to imagine the numerals beyond the periphery of your sight.

Sitting comfortably, begin to deep breathe. Now, without moving the head, look directly upward as high as possible, searching for the number twelve at the top center of the clock face. Once you have "seen" it, move the eyes slowly to the right and locate the numeral one. Deep breathing in and out, go on to two, and then to three. Move the eyes very slowly.

At this point, return your eyes to the center of the clock and then close the lids. Gently place the heels of your hands over the closed eyes and hold them there a moment. Allow the feeling of warmth to be transmitted from your hands to your lids.

Remove your hands and allow your eyes to swing to the right in search of the numeral four on the imagined clock face. Move slowly on to five, and then to six, deep breathing all the while. At six, return the eyes to the center of the imagined timepiece and repeat the palming method of placing your hands across the closed lids.

Continue on around the face of the clock, pausing at nine for the palming and again at twelve. After resting for awhile, repeat this exercise in reverse. That is, start at twelve o'clock, swing leftward to eleven and on to ten and so on, in a counter-clockwise pattern. Combine deep breathing with the eye movements in order to supply an increased amount of oxygen to your body during the exercises.

After a week or two of practicing these eye movements, you may begin on a second set of exercises. By now, if you've practiced daily with the rotating movements following the clock numerals, your eye muscles should be somewhat strengthened and ready for the Point-Counter-Point movements.

Sitting in a relaxed easy pose as with the previous exercises, deep breathing in and out, find the numeral one on the face of the imagined oversize clock. Remember to look upward as high as your vision will take you, but without moving the head. Now, without pause, swing your eyes downward toward seven o'clock. Close the eyes and use the palming method of placing the heels of the hands against the eyes. Now, removing the hands, swing the eyes upward to find eleven on the clock face, and move down to five. Repeat the palming technique.

After this, you would find ten and four, and two and eight, employing the palming of the eyes for relaxation after each set of numbers, and combining deep breathing with the eye movements.

Daily eye exercises can help to restore weakened vision while serving as a means of relaxation at the same time.

Neck and Throat Exercises

It is this part of the body that can betray a woman who has concentrated on all the requirements of beauty except that of tone. The neck and throat area is quick to bespeak weight loss or gain, neglected treatment, or tension which causes unsightly cords to stand out.

The way one holds the head is dependent to a degree on the condition and strength of one's neck muscles. If the slender foundation on which the head rests is underexercised, there cannot be the erect posture that shows zest and enthusiasm for living. In fact, this one area of weakness alone can lead to other more serious ones. When the

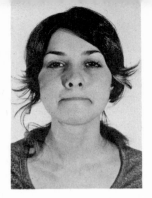

head is not held upright, but is allowed to slant forward, the shoulders in turn are pulled out of line and rounded. This enforced curving of the spinal area breeds its own discomforts and ailments.

While the neck exercises in Chapter Three are a necessary part of regaining and maintaining health in this area, the following practices using the throat muscles tend strongly to eliminate sagging tissue and double chins.

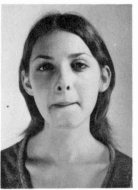

Standing or sitting, hold the shoulders erect and the spine upright. Very slowly thrust the lower lip up over the upper lip as high as it will go. Hold it in place a moment, relax, and try it again.

Now roll the lower lip inward toward the opened mouth, tucking the upper lip downward as far as it will reach. Practice opening and closing the mouth as the lower lip keeps rolling inward and the upper lip keeps reaching for the chin. Do this ten to twenty times a day for tone. Though this is a gentle action, you can feel the tightening of the flesh under the chin each time you roll the lip inward if you touch it with your fingers.

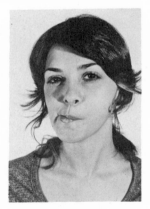

In another movement, keep the lips closed and move them as far to the right as possible. Relax and then move them to the left. Now, in an easy action move them both back and forth several times.

Visualize the extreme downward turn of the drama mask of tragedy. Mimic this with a downward force of the lip corners.

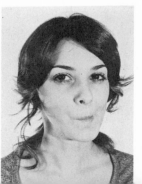

Bust Development

The concern about bust measurements in this country exceeds that in any other. Fashion had its sweater girls in the forties, but following that, there was an emphasis on the flat chested woman of chic. Even more recent is the fashion edict of wearing no support whatsoever, and creating a "free" appearance for this part of the body.

There should be a natural comfort to the body at all times, and this can come about if the breast area is kept as firm as possible, no matter what the current style. One of the finest firming exercises for the breast is gained by practicing the Hand Greeting in Chapter 6 and the Cowhead Pose in Chapter 12. The pull on the pectoral muscles around the breast develops tone and strengthens the muscles. Another beneficial posture is that of the Yoga Mudra in Chapter 7. Any of the exercises that use the upper portion of the body should be helpful in gaining and maintaining a healthy firmness to the chest area. Posture, too, is of the greatest importance in preventing premature sagging of the breasts.

A means of reducing flabbiness and regaining a lithe bust line is found in practicing the Blade. This movement pulls the arms and shoulders backward and flexes the pectoral muscles, bringing increased tone and resiliency

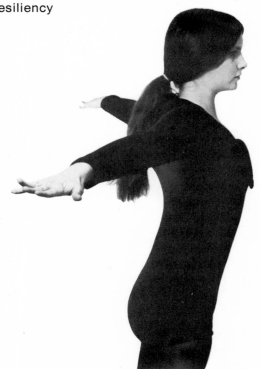

The Blade—
Exercise I

Standing in an upright position with the spinal column held erectly, extend the arms directly out sideways from the shoulder. Squeeze inward with the shoulder blades as tightly as possible, without moving the arms at all. You should be able to feel the pull on the entire upper area of your body. Deep breathe in and out while practicing this pose.

EXERCISES FOR THE SPECIFIC AREAS

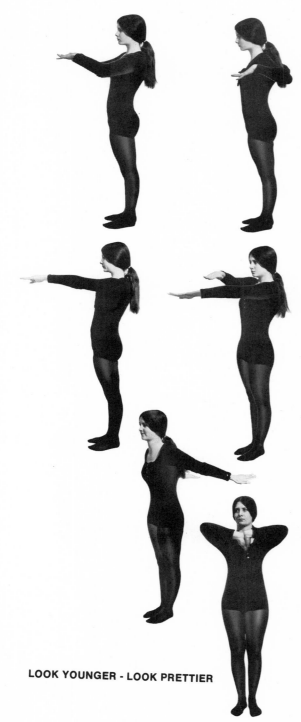

Exercise II

An exercise for firming the bust line that can be practiced at odd moments in the office or at home also relieves tension of the neck area, since a massaging action is felt here, too, during the Elbow-Bend.

Sitting or standing with the spine in an upright position, take a deep breath and extend the arms in a straight line before you to the front. Exhale slowly as you pull the arms in a diamond-shaped position backward until the elbows are behind the shoulders and the hands are beside the breasts. Relax and repeat this movement several times.

Exercise III

In another position, stand with the arms at shoulder level directly in front of the body with the palms facing downward. Taking a deep breath, slowly bring the hands toward each other, palms remaining downward. Allow the right hand and arm to pass under the left one until there is a cross formed at the elbows. Separate the arms and move them in an opposite direction behind the shoulders as far as possible. Return the arms slowly to the front and repeat.

Exercise IV

Standing or sitting upright with the spine held erectly, place the palms of the hand together in a prayer position before the chest. Very slowly turn the ends of the fingers toward the chest and continue on downward with them as far as you can turn them.

Repeat several times.

LOOK YOUNGER - LOOK PRETTIER

Swayback

The off-balance posture that either creates or encourages the hollow stance position of the back can usually be eliminated with discipline and corrective exercises. Presenting an awkward appearance, the hollowed or swayed back creates the secondary grievance of a forward-thrust stomach.

Those afflicted with this extreme posture generally walk on the heels rather than the balls of the feet, as is correct. This improper placement of weight onto the heels throws the body off balance, and to compensate for this manner of tipping backward, the stomach is thrust forward.

Such abnormal hollowing of the back can be effectively dealt with by the use of the following exercises, practiced daily.

To begin the correcting of this poor posture that can lead to malfunctioning of the internal organs if left unchecked, there must be daily barefoot practice in order to restore normal balance to the body. During every practice session, stand as straight as possible. Now roll your weight from your heels onto the balls of your feet. You should immediately feel a shifting of weight and a straightening of the body. If performed correctly, your body will be in alignment now. Practice this rolling forward at different times during the day until the practice becomes routine habit.

In order to strengthen the weak back muscles that have either resulted from or helped create this condition in the first place, exercises are in order. Lying comfortably flat on the floor on your back and in loose clothing, raise the right knee toward the body and bring it back as close to the chest as possible, simultaneously flinging both of your arms behind your head to touch the floor.

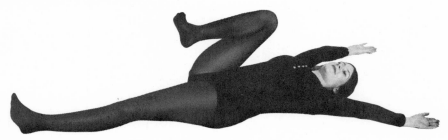

Repeat the exercise using the left leg and both arms.

The Head-to-Knee movement in Chapter 3 is also excellent for strengthening the swayed back. However, care must be taken not to impose a strain on the weakened area. Do not press forward in this position. Go only as far as you comfortably can. Daily exercise will gradually limber the spine to the point that you can manage the complete movement without harm to your body.

The Hands - Easy Exercises For Arthritic Hands and Fingers

The hands carry a burden of work and expression throughout their existence. They are one's silent servants, and it is usually not until their degree of performance is lessened that true awareness of their importance comes. The hands in their irreplaceable usefulness are an extension of the mind.

Why, then, should one permit the hands to become disabled from lack of use, or through crippling arthritis, which, if it cannot be avoided, can be halted enough to permit continued usage of the hands and fingers.

When the calcium deposits that create the knobbed, deformed characteristics appear, the natural tendency is to avoid the pain that comes from moving the swollen joints. In time, because of the stiffness coming both from the calcium deposits and the lack of movement, the hands can become mere appendages without any real use.

Yoga teaches that exercising the body and the hands will help ward off the painful effects of this disease. The Hand-Spread is an effective means of gaining and maintaining full use of this part of the body.

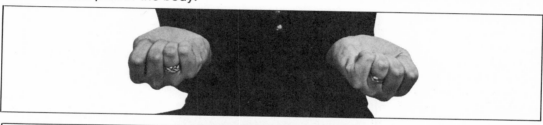

Exercise I

Hold the hands in tight balls before you. With the fingers turned into the palms and the thumb tucked behind the fingers, slowly release the fingers, taking a minimum of thirty seconds to do so. Slowly thrust the fingers and thumbs outward into a stiffened fan-shaped gesture, stretching them as far as they will go.

Allow the spread hand and palm to remain in this widely opened position for the same length of time it took to open the hand. Then relax both fingers and hands and slowly return the fingers to their ball-shaped position. Repeat this exercise at least ten times daily, very slowly.

For those with severe limitations in hand and finger usage, begin more slowly, and practice fewer times a day until there is complete comfort in performance before working up to ten times. Practicing this exercise slowly will bring far more rewards than a hasty performance. The slowness accustoms the hands to movement, and makes the exercise less painful and more acceptable as agility returns to the area.

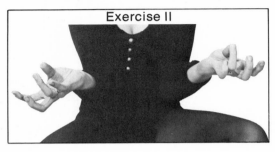

Exercise II

With the hands spread wide, palms held upward, press the tip of the thumb against each of the tips of the four fingers. Do this slowly and press with as much strength as you have. You will notice a quick surge of blood brought to the fingertips by the stimulation. This exercise is also beneficial to healthy fingernail growth.

Exercises For Strengthening Weak Ankles

Sureness of foot, excellent posture, and correction of many figure faults can be brought about by strengthening weak ankles. After all, if the foundation of a building is not sturdy enough to support the structure, there should be no surprise that the building is bowed, bent, or otherwise faulty in appearance.

The same rule would apply to our own bodies. If one cannot support one's spinal column in a straight posture, then hollow chest, rounded back and shoulders, and other unhealthy conditions develop. In order to gain the needed strength to carry one's poundage, here is a good exercise for strengthening the ankles.

Exercise I

Lie on the floor on your back with the arms by the side. First lift the right foot a few inches above the floor and describe a circle very slowly, five times. Bring the right foot down and relax. Now repeat the exercise with the left foot, and relax.

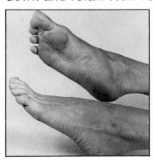 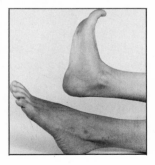 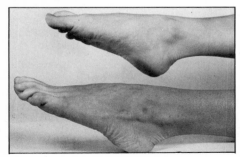

EXERCISES FOR SPECIFIC AREAS

Exercise II

Sit upright and try to bring the soles of the feet together so they are heel to heel and toe to toe.

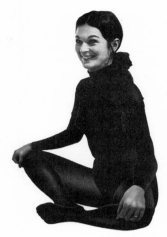

Exercise III

Standing in an upright position with the arms straight before you on a level with your eyes, slowly swing around to the right as far as your arms will take you. Hold the feet flat on the floor without permitting them to move. There is a tendency for the feet to swing around with the arms, but in restraining this action, the ankles are strengthened by the play brought to bear in this area.

Now reverse the direction and slowly swing around to the left. Repeat this exercise several times in both directions.

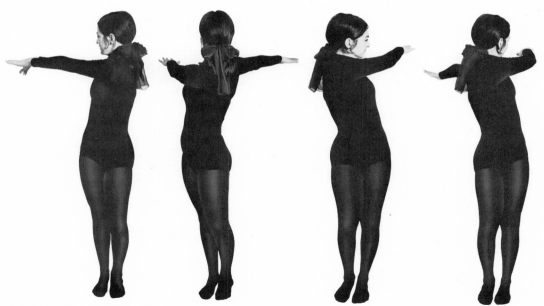

LOOK YOUNGER - LOOK PRETTIER

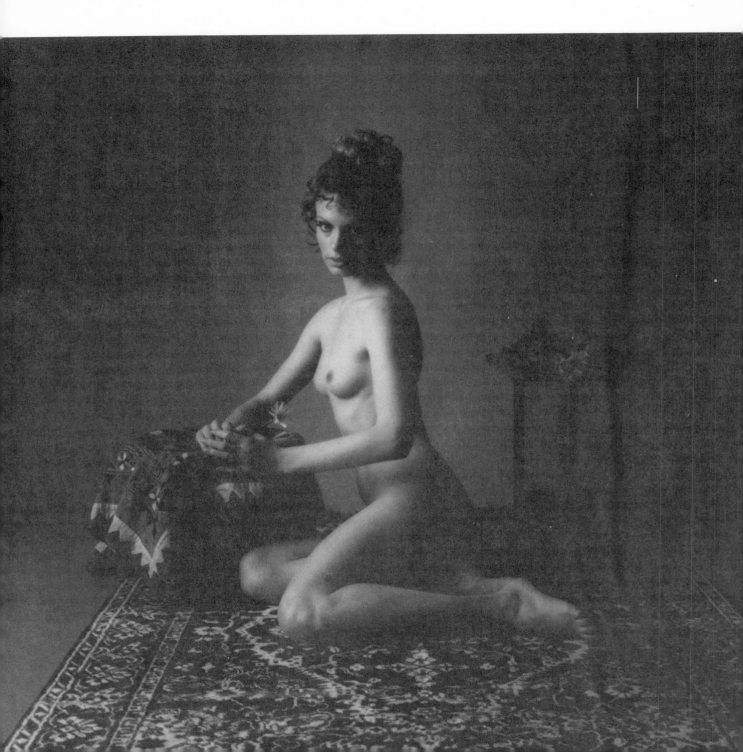

CHAPTER FOURTEEN - A BEAUTIFUL BODY IS A CLEAN BODY

In order to cleanse the body of wastes that accumulate daily, four main channels serve as disposal organs. The skin, the lungs, the kidneys, and the intestines carry away the debris that the body casts off as poisons.

Too often one may think of only one or two organs as being used in this capacity. And while the intestines and kidneys are vitally important, the skin (the largest organ of the body) and the lungs carry a heavy burden of responsibility, too.

Beauty and health cannot be had if any one of the four disposal organs are sluggish or otherwise poorly working. If the pores in the skin are not kept open and clean, resultant misery emerges as clogged skin develops infections from hardened oil and dead cells.

Good nutrition is as important to the external appearance of the skin as it is to the internal upkeep of the body. The need for foods that nourish and provide cleansing action to the intestines can be compared to the need to prepare a house for a painting operation that will beautify it. When the basic structure is sound and kept in good repair, the overall upkeep is kept to a minimum.

There is no use applying a pretty covering to scaling, faulty walls. No amount of outside decor will long conceal the rot that has set in on once sturdy materials. To try to conceal a muddy complexion and blemishes with a layer of makeup is as foolish as to try to cover peeling walls with a fresh coat of paint.

In both cases, the action is a waste of time and effort. To paint a flaking building will merely add to the mottled appearance. A coat of make-up over a blemished complexion will congest the area further and make the clearing up all the more difficult.

For a first-rate improvement of the skin, start from within with a plan for internal cleansing. While you are feeding the body its healing and beautifying foods, begin to work on the skin itself.

Plan an overall program of deep cleansing to allow the breath of life to pour in, and the necessary waste materials to be lifted out. While it is not glamorous to think of the skin as an organ of disposal, it is just that, and performs that function most admirably when permitted.

Our job is to see that nothing interferes with this task. Every pore must be kept open. Firm skin tone must be sought. Fresh air must be given the skin at frequent intervals, both by external methods of exposure and internally by deep breathing in order to supply the bloodstream with purifying oxygen.

There are many methods of cleansing the skin. First and foremost, there is the internal method of consuming sufficient fresh fruits and vegetables. This promotes proper waste disposal through other organs. It also conditions the skin and helps prevent the collapse or slowdown of cellular growth.

External methods of cleansing the skin offer a varied means of sweeping away the debris. One of the most effective skin-cleansing methods involves the use of a complexion brush. These soft-bristled brushes enter each and every pore and help to break up and sweep out accumulated oils and dead tissues. After such a cleansing, several rinses in warm and then cool water will remove the soap. Make sure the final rinse is with an apple-cider-and-water solution which restores the acid mantle native to the body. Then pat the skin dry.

Another means of cleansing the skin is to use a sponge made of marine life. This firm scrubber will rub away dead cells and expose living skin that must breathe in order to be healthy. This sponge is nothing more than the natural sponge that we use, for instance, for cleaning our car.

Facials that stimulate by bringing a fresh blood supply can also carry away accumulated waste matter from the skin. A fresh strawberry facial will cut through the embedded pore oils and float out the collected wastes. Quick facials can be had merely by rubbing a washed, unsprayed strawberry over the entire facial surface, allowing it to remain on for five to ten minutes and then rinsing this off. Any other acid-type fruit will serve well, too.

The Lungs

The lungs carry out their twofold purpose by bringing in quantities of oxygen and channelling out the waste products of carbon dioxide and other gaseous impurities thrown off by the body. In healthy lungs, there is an even exchange of waste for oxygen which enables the body to function.

If the breathing is shallow and of scanty supply, obviously there will not be an even oxygen-waste exchange, and the impurities will not be removed from the body. Just as important, if exhalation, about which one seldom thinks, is indifferent and weak, even an adequate amount of indrawn oxygen cannot be utilized, for it is not until the lungs are relieved of stagnant air that fresh air can permeate them and enter the bloodstream.

A BEAUTIFUL BODY IS A CLEAN BODY

It is in these instances that the Lion exercise becomes invaluable. The forceful expulsion of breath while practicing the Lion drives the gaseous impurities of the bloodstream from the lower lung extremities, permitting the immediate acceptance of fresh air.

When breathing is shallow, and is done through a tightened chest action that does not permit an easy flow of air, the lungs cannot perform their duty well. Poor posture, long hours in overheated rooms, and little physical exercise will also exact their toll in lung performance. When neglected, the internal airways of the body can become polluted as easily as can the atmosphere around us.

It is for this reason that one should go for a brisk walk and indulge in deep breathing. The fresh oxygen supply acts as an internal bath, rinsing the bloodstream of accumulated poisonous gases. One also wisely turns to Yoga exercises in order to achieve maximum lung performance.

It is for this reason that all Yoga exercises are performed with deep-breathing techniques. As the body moves and stretches itself in an asana, a greater supply of oxygen is pushed along to the furthest reaches of the body, and especially to those areas of the lungs that have been neglected.

The Kidneys

From our earliest days we have been told of the value of drinking six to eight glasses of water daily. But frankly this practice cannot be easily maintained. Either we don't like the taste of water, or else find it inconvenient to establish this daily practice.

An effective method of water-drinking may be created by placing six or eight pennies on the right-hand side of the sink. Each time you go near the sink, drink a glass of water and place one penny on the opposite side of the sink. Continue this practice throughout the day, and by evening, the water will have been consumed and all the pennies will be on the left side of the sink. Leave them there, and the following morning begin again this serious game of flushing out the body. Only this time the pennies will go one by one to the right side of the sink.

This eliminates forgetfulness, mistakes in counting, and helps to achieve inner cleanliness. But the liquid consumed in this practice must be water. Coffee, tea, soft drinks or other liquids cannot be considered the same as water.

The water should be taken between meals, rather than accompanying them, in order to avoid diluting the digestive juices needed during and following mealtime.

The use of the following is considered beneficial for the kidneys:

Sage tea	Barley	Watercress
Juniper berry tea	Parsley	Asparagus
Alfalfa tea or sprouts		

The Intestines

In order to have a beautiful and healthy body, cleanliness of the inner organs is vital. One's entire sense of well-being and one's outward appearance are dependent on the degree to which one disposes of waste materials. When there is inadequate exercise and poor nutrition, clogging of the intestines ensues. The outer skin will immediately show the results of this faulty elimination. Impurities held within the body will thrust outward in the form of poor skin conditions, outbreaks of boils, abscesses and other scar-producing afflictions.

Diseases can easily begin from accumulated toxins that have piled up within the neglected body. Wastes that are not removed lodge within, and putrefaction sets in. Premature aging of the body, including the skin, is speeded along by a lack of inner cleansing.

Many persons who would not consider going out with spotted, soiled clothing and who are immaculate in dress, nevertheless have intestines burdened with putrefactive matter and a bloodstream that is sewerous in condition. It is far wiser to concentrate on this hidden part of the body than to be concerned with the outer facade. The inner condition will determine the appearance of the external.

Beauty demands a certain routine, and will not settle for less. There must be a regular, active movement of the body in order to stimulate action in the intestines and to keep them toned for action. Sedentary living will not bring about health and beauty. Merely walking about one's daily chores will not do it either, for this is not enough physical movement. And it is not scientific. There has to be planned, daily, physical activity in order to move food wastes along and to prevent the development of lazy intestines.

The same six or eight glasses of water that aid the kidneys in flushing out impurities will also loosen the solid matter in the intestines and prevent accumulations of hardened wastes.

Food can be chosen in order to correct and maintain a healthy elimination. This desirable state cannot be had with indifferent nutrition. In earlier days, it was easier to remain healthy. Our foods were less diverse, but they were pure foods, and not products created to stimulate taste buds only. Grains were whole and complete, vegetables were fresh and packed with natural food value. Meats, fish and poultry were untainted with chemical treatments.

Today, the partly artificial food we pass on as nourishment to our bodies, helps bring about the toxic condition that causes poisonous wastes to lie within. In the healthy body there is a constant wave-like motion along the entire length of the alimentary canal. This movement propels food along its course until it is properly digested, nutrients are absorbed, and waste sent on to the bowels for elimination. This is known as peristaltic action, and if it fails to operate properly, then the food, either partially or poorly digested,

A BEAUTIFUL BODY IS A CLEAN BODY

does not get moved along, and in consequence remains to clog the intestines and become toxic. When the poisonous wastes remain in the body, the area becomes a breeding ground for disease.

Because modern devitalized foods slow down the proper working of the intestines and bring discomfort in the resultant congestion, the average person turns to the use of laxatives as a means of ridding his body of this waste matter. Millions of dollars a year are spent on laxatives and purges in an attempt to cleanse the inner organs of the results of the soft, processed, nonfoods that lie inert in the system.

Laxatives are habit-forming, and with their continued usage, the intestines lose their tone. There is no longer the easy peristaltic action that in a healthy body automatically takes care of elimination without any artificial help.

Both longevity and beauty are associated with the degree of cleanliness existing in the intestinal tract. There can be no real enthusiasm for living, either, if the channels of elimination are clogged, and the body is forced to deal with both today's fuel and yesterday's rubbish. Indifference and neglect of these body functions will exact a heavy toll. Until one has the body in prime working order through exercise and good nutrition, one cannot expect to enjoy life to its fullest.

Correcting faulty elimination is not a difficult matter. Yet this affliction is a spectre in the Western world where we dote on soft beds, soft chairs, soft foods, and convenient transportation. Though faulty elimination can be cleared up at any age, preventive methods should commence during the earliest years. Car pools to transport children could become walking pools (with the same chaperonage to ensure the child's safety) designed to accustom the child to walking reasonable distances.

This practice could continue throughout the school years, and carry on as one enters a career. Instead of the usual bus ride to work, one could use a bicycle for practical distances. Or, if necessary, drive part way, and cycle the rest.

In addition to increasing the amount of physical movement in one's day, one should carefully examine his eating habits. Instead of a quick lunch at some counter restaurant, the midday meal could be used to supply a large amount of the day's nutrition if one prepared the food at home from fresh vegetables, fruits and protein-supplying meats or cheeses.

Much of the distress of faulty elimination can be corrected by changing one's diet. We should turn from all-white flour and its products, white sugar, and white rice, and replace these non-foods with whole grains, and either raw sugar or honey for sweetening. This would help correct some of the worst cases of constipation. We would also do well to forego all soft drinks and fried foods.

Once these steps are taken, one should start adding foods of value to the diet. One will immediately note the new ease of the eliminative process. Add a juicy, unwaxed apple daily to your diet. Have at least one large, raw salad composed of dark-leaf lettuce, of the romaine, chickory, or curley endive variety. Add a grated carrot, diced celery, radishes, green pepper and tomato to the bowl. For dressing, avoid the pudding-type "Russian" sauces. Instead, sprinkle the juice of half a lemon or a tablespoon or two of apple cider vinegar over the leaves and then pour any cold-pressed vegetable or nut oil over the salad.

Stewed dried fruits for breakfast are another aid to developing healthy intestines. Starting the day with steel-cut or old fashioned oatmeal supplies the body with the B vitamins so necessary to good intestinal health. Other helps in the diet include the use of molasses, whey, raisins (soaked overnight in water and eaten before breakfast), a teaspoon of cold pressed nut or vegetable oil daily in the diet, a cup of warm water and the juice of one half a lemon taken thirty minutes before breakfast, yogurt taken daily, and one tablespoon of brewer's yeast dissolved in water or juice, and taken three times a day.

EXERCISES FOR ELIMINATION

Exercise I

Sit with the buttocks on the heels and the arms loosely held over the lower part of the abdomen. The back of the arms and hands will be resting atop the lap at the conjunction of the thighs and abdomen. Take a deep breath and exhale slowly as you lower the head to the floor. Do not permit the buttocks to leave their position on the heels. Return to an upright sitting position, relax, and repeat this movement several times, very slowly, remembering to deep breathe in and out.

Exercise II

Laying flat on the back on the floor with the arms by the side, commence breathing deeply in and out. Now, on an in-drawn breath, reach for the knee of the right leg and bring it up to the chest and then exhale. Return the leg to a prone position. Repeat the exercise with the left leg. Relax, deep breathe and bring both knees upward toward the chest. Exhale and return the legs to their prone position on the floor. Repeat this exercise several times.

For rewarding benefits, both exercises should be performed upon arising in the morning.

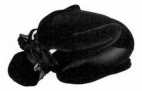

A BEAUTIFUL BODY IS A CLEAN BODY

The Tongue

Along with the major channels of elimination, there is one additional area that should be acknowledged as doing its part to rid the body of waste materials, though it would not be considered a major disposal organ. Nevertheless, Yoga feels that the tongue is too often ignored when an effort is made to assist the body in waste removal.

Usually we think of the mouth as an intake for food, without being greatly concerned as to its daily cleansing other than the usual brushing of the teeth. Too often the tongue goes uncleansed and provides a ready harbor for wastes.

Yoga believes that it is just as essential to maintain hygienic conditions with reference to the tongue as elsewhere. It is not difficult to remove the accumulations on that organ, and if you inspect this part of the mouth, you may be surprised at what you see.

Examine the tongue upon awakening in the morning. Note the residue of mucus or film coating this area. Now, with the handle of a spoon turned sideways, carefully scrape it down the length of the tongue, starting from the back. Note the slimy residue that has coated your tongue overnight. After removing the film, rinse the mouth thoroughly and then examine the pink evidence of a cleansed tongue.

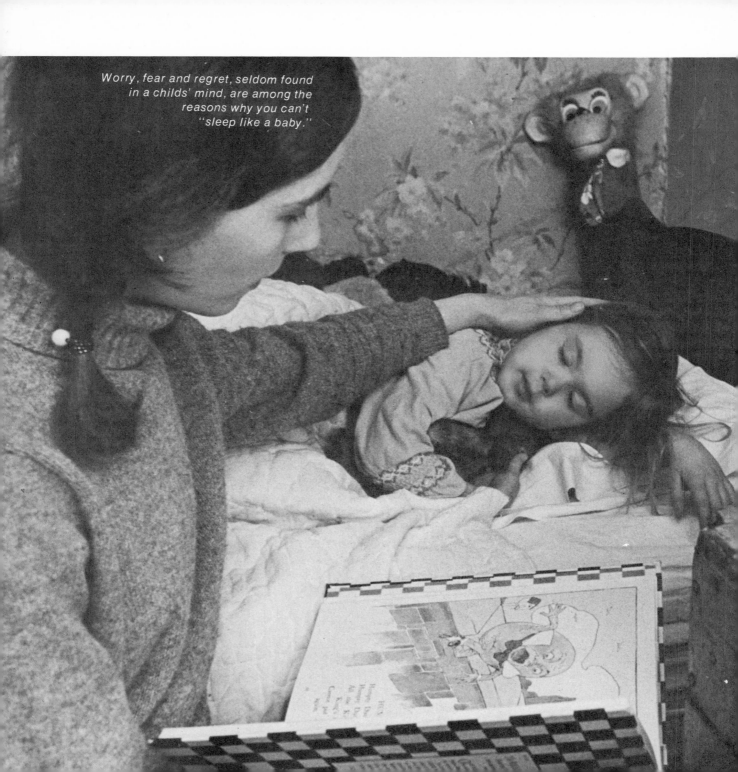

Worry, fear and regret, seldom found in a childs' mind, are among the reasons why you can't "sleep like a baby."

CHAPTER FIFTEEN - RELAX YOUR WAY TO SOUND SLEEP

Sleeplessness has become a major malady in the modern world. The tensions and drives that structure the day for many, linger and create a turbulent atmosphere during the night. Restless minds review the day's activities, and jangled nerves deny sleep to the exhausted body.

A tense, taut body and mind are not going to yield to mental suggestion, or even to a command, to go to sleep, merely because one's schedule orders it. A distressed mind and body have no clock and no schedule. If they have been mistreated, they cannot respond to nature's laws, which require an amount of time for repair and restoration.

The body at sleep may be compared to a rehabilitation factory. It is here, during the off hours, that the body is soothed and repaired and made ready for another day's living. Though creative thought processes are halted during the period of sleep, within the complex body and mind there are facilities for complete restoration. Sleep is not a cataleptic state; muscles do flex as they drift into a state of complete relaxation, and regular movements throughout the night help the body to achieve a maximum of comfortable rest.

But this is possible only in the body that does not pursue its battles on a twenty-four-hour-a-day basis.

A man may achieve his highest material goals, taste all the worldly successes he desires, and list among his accomplishments impressive deeds. Yet if he is among the millions of insomniacs, he would many times trade his cherished possessions and abilities for the unconscious state that rests and refurbishes his mind and body.

The elusiveness of sleep has been discussed, and remedies sought, probably as long as man has had a restless mind and turbulent emotions. Certainly, there are enough recipes for suggested cures of this affliction to suggest that it is a problem of vast proportions.

Detailed volumes have been written on the subject, and the whys and wherefores of the sleepless state explored page after page. Some of the books offer sensible advice, while others merely repeat statistics and complicated theories and practices that exhaust one without proving to be practical. There are pieces of equipment designed to lull a resistant body into a soporific state, beds that vibrate, eye masks that shut out the light, and earplugs that close off the sounds of the noisy world.

How much of all this is successful depends on the person involved and his particular problem. Some persons have grown so desperate that they have resorted to being hypnotized in the hopes of sidetracking the cause of their sleeplessness. But learning to thwart insomnia is not enough. The body cannot exist in its best state on contrived practices.

Who are the sleepless ones? Certainly not a person of serenity and composure. Neither is it one who has concerned himself with his body and catered to it by supplying it with the right materials to perform. A person deeply involved in some gratifying service to mankind, which in turn brings contentment to himself, would hardly be troubled with sleeplessness.

An insomniac might be anyone who does not have strict control over his own body. The hasty person, the impulsive type, and the brooder usually are prone to the wakeful state. Worries that begin in the morning and are nurtured throughout the day will seldom be relinquished just because the body is placed in a prone position at night.

The quick-tempered person is another potential insomniac. By day, hasty words are spoken, and by night the price for quick anger is paid in regret. But merely going without sleep as a guilt payment for one's harsh words will not cure this type of insomnia. As a matter of fact, many persons of this flash-like temperament use the method of guilt and punishment to balance out a day. But the price is a high one, and habit becomes addiction.

By far the greater number of insomniacs count among their causes for sleeplessness feelings of worry, fear, and regret. Few emotions are left out of the causes listed for a sleepless state. Once a pattern has been established, the body seems to accept the routine through which it writhes hour after hour. Sometimes physical exhaustion will rescue the mind and dull its dervish-like dartings. Sometimes one is not so fortunate, and morning will come without an appreciable amount of sleep having been had throughout the night.

These self-destructive forces must be dispelled if one is to be able to perform one's daily tasks efficiently. They cannot be permanently and successfully exorcised by tranquilizers, sleeping tablets, or any other drug or alcohol.

Of course, there is the temporary type of sleeplessness which does not bring with it the cause for concern of the more entrenched type. Any unusual news of an exciting or disruptive nature can be so stimulating or distressing that the body is momentarily thrown into a state of turmoil. Until the mind makes peace with the body by accepting or rejecting the disturbance, sleep will be elusive.

Another major cause of sleeplessness stems from an underexercised body - going about one's daily tasks seldom insures sufficient movement and flexing of the body. Exhaustion can come from a regular, sedentary schedule of little or no activity. But this type of fatigue is more apt to cause one to thrash about the bed with wide-open eyes. And this type of weariness speaks of a protesting body, of muscles and ligaments grown toneless. By refusing to relax, the physical body thrusts its condition onto the mental.

But by teaching one to overcome the physical tensions of a sedentary existence, yoga can bring mental composure. Once the mind is freed of physical irritations, it can relax and direct calming thoughts to all parts of the body.

From the moment an insomniac starts to practice Hatha Yoga, with the physical exercises listed in detail in this book, he is on a path to healthful sleep. From the first roll of his body on the floor, the sleepless person has turned to a method that has brought sleep to thousands and thousands of persons.

In addition to the soothing of tautened body muscles, there should be a slowing down of uncontrolled mental processes. The mind of an insomniac darts here and there, examining first one set of thoughts and then another. And having resolved nothing, his mind will flit back again and again to the distressing problem. The release from worry, concern, fear, and other emotions will help to bring the insomniac to tranquility and sleep.

The practice of deep breathing with Yoga exercises is especially helpful in preparing for sleep. The indrawn quantities of oxygen will help to soothe the body, relax it, and restore it to a composure that is conducive to sleep. Tensed-up muscles can be deterrent enough to ward off sleep for hours. The act of breathing deeply in and out slows down the body mechanism running full tilt from anxieties. Just as you would employ deep breathing to calm your nerves during a confrontation in the daytime, so you should use the same device for achieving sleep. Gradually, the deep breathing is relinquished in sleep preparation until the breathing returns to normal.

Nature's Sleep Pattern

Yoga says the best sleep pattern is that of following the sun, as in nature. This method of early retirement would suggest that the sleeping habits of many in our Western society are very poor, especially in the case of those who stay up until late hours and then sleep late the following morning.

Since most animal and plant life goes to rest at sundown and comes to life with the sun's rising the following morning, this would seem a more natural approach to regular sleeping habits.

The early morning hours are important because the air is fresh, and also because there is true quiet at this time that is difficult to know at any other period of the day. Those who practice early rising say they gain a measure of tranquility and preparation that can carry them through the more hectic hours later in the day. While it would prove difficult and impractical for many to try to observe this ancient method of living and sleeping, nevertheless the pattern that is the more natural or closer to the habits of nature, is usually the more beneficial.

Individual Requirements For Sleep

While the individual requirements for sleep vary, the healthy body generally needs between six and eight hours a night to rest and restore itself. Unless the body is in excellent physical condition, six hours may prove too few. Sometimes exhaustion is so acute that even without any emotional distress, complete relaxation will not come in sleep. In these cases, usually accompanied by taut muscles, it is far better to leave the bed and perform a few Yoga exercises. Instead of making one more exhausted, and therefore, more wide awake, these movements will gently work at the tight, rebellious body muscles and harried mind to release them gradually from tension's paralyzing hold. Sometimes after less than five minutes of the Rock and Roll or the Swan or any other easy movement, one can return to bed and find immediate relief in the form of natural sleep.

Yoga teaches another method of gaining complete relaxation in preparation for sleep. This practice can be carried on at home prior to retiring each night, in order to put the body in a proper framework of total and complete relaxation. It is not a form of hypnosis, but instead, it is a method of the mind gaining control over the physical body.

The gentle commands of the Total Relaxation exercise gradually subdue the resistant body and in a few brief minutes the entire body seems to be floating free of heavy emotions and tensions.

The mind, by gaining control of the body, assumes its rightful position as commander of the body. Once in charge, with no resistance from a clamoring body that aches from tightly held muscles, the mind produces serenity. With the combination of a relaxed body and a soothed mind, sleep comes quickly.

Total relaxation is beneficial when performed at the end of each Yoga practice of the day. After one or two lessons, with someone reading the following directions aloud, it is possible to use this technique to gain peace and to become relaxed without additional supervision. It is a simple, but effective practice.

Total Relaxation

Lie with the back flat on the floor. Place the arms comfortably by the sides. Separate the feet slightly and relax them. Now take several deep breaths, in and out, very slowly. As each part of the body is called into action, allow it to relax. There must be no short-cuts. Concentrate on each of the following words as they are read aloud and obey them:

Close the eyes and relax the body from the toes upward. Try to relax the entire face. Let the toes relax. Allow the feet to be apart and to find a comfortable slant. Relax the ankles. Relax the calves. Relax the knees. Relax the thighs. Relax the hips. Relax the waist. Relax the chest.

Relax the shoulders. Allow the arms to relax. Relax the elbows. Relax the wrists. Allow the hands to relax. Let the fingers separate and relax them. Relax the back. Relax the neck. Relax the head. Release the scalp and allow it to relax. Relax the forehead. Relax the eyes. Relax the nose. Relax the cheeks.

Separate the lips slightly and relax them. Let the chin relax. Allow the entire body to sink into the floor.

Forget all the worries of your life. Forget the things you have to do and the things you want to do. These plans have no part of you at the moment. You are freed of all worries and concerns. Think only of the deep peace and relaxation you now know.

Feel the body getting very light. Visualize a fleecy white cloud drifting along in the sky. Watch it move slowly through the open space. Think of yourself as a cloud, slowly, gently drifting so peacefully through the beautiful sky, feeling no weight.

Drift in this fashion for several minutes. Then slowly stretch the entire body. Now, without any haste, rise to a sitting position.

This Total Relaxation will prepare both body and mind for sleep. General preparations for retiring should have been completed prior to this practice so one can go directly to bed, and so to sleep. If the directions are followed carefully, then the entire body will be receptive to normal and natural sleep.

For some, a different imagined scene is more conducive to tranquility. In this matter you must choose the more harmonious setting as your peace promoter. Perhaps a seashore scene with gently rolling waves will form the background for your relaxation exercise. The aim is to establish in one's mind the background that speaks of tranquility. A lake scene, a field of golden grain or miles of forest solitude will please many. Be individual in your selection.

Total Relaxation is Helpful at Other Times

One does not have to wait until bedtime to put this highly successful relaxation method to use. It can be part of a daytime plan, also. If you are at a desk, or wherever your workday might take you, some parts of the formula can be applied to good advantage.

Naturally, you would not attempt the complete formula when you are driving a car. Instead, you would limit yourself to relaxing the shoulder and the neck area.

While Yoga teaches that complete relaxation of the body will serve to overcome insomnia, there are some additional methods that can be used in searching for sleep. Some of these suggestions are quite old, and have come down through time accompanied by praise as to their effectiveness. Since these are all harmless remedies and many times give soothing results, one can try them until a favorite is found.

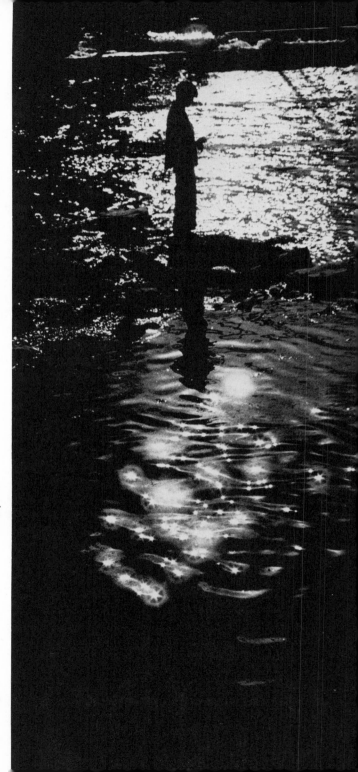

Visualize a tranquil scene and let it dominate your thinking. Forget your worries and things you want to do. Relax.

Old Fashioned Remedies For Sleeplessness

Honey and Lemon Soother: Squeeze the juice of one half a lemon into a glass of hot water. Mix in two tablespoons of raw honey. Mix well and sip slowly thirty minutes before retiring.

Lettuce has long been considered to be a sedative that will bring a natural, unlabored sleep, free from any side effects. Eating several green leaves of any variety except iceberg lettuce quiets the nerves. Or chop finely several of the darker leaves into a cup of water and simmer this atop a burner for two or three minutes. Strain and drink this lettuce tea while it is lukewarm, and immediately before retiring.

An insomniac cure known and used in many parts of the world is as old as the apple itself. A mixture of two teaspoons of raw honey and two teaspoons of apple-cider vinegar and a glass of warm water is supposed to bring sleep soon after taking the solution.

Camomile tea relaxes the body and prepares it for sleep, and has been in use for several centuries.

If you have a safe sleeping area either on a porch, balcony, or anywhere in the open, sleep is more likely to come to the distressed body and mind. In temperate climates this is practical much of the year around. In colder regions, only the warmer months can be used for this refreshingly natural way of falling asleep. A cot or hammock will serve very well, along with sufficient cover to ward off the chill of night hours.

There is something basic and splendid found in sleeping under an open sky. No one tosses and turns when he is bedded down on a level with pine needles. Sleep seems to be almost instantaneous when one lies down at night with the scent of birch, pine and earth all brewed together and served as a scented nightcap of air.

Sleep with your head pointing north and your feet pointing south. This places your body in a line with the earth's magnetic current. The magnetic pull on the body which is lying counter to the current has created insomnia in some people. It is simple enough to turn one's bed with the head facing the north and the feet facing the south, just to be on the safe side, even if you do not accept the theory.

The use of the skin brush for insomnia is an old European custom. Advocates of the system say that it clears the body's pores for breathing by removing the suffocating mantle of dead cells, and gently relaxes the body while it readies it for blissful sleep. All pharmacy and department stores in France sell the rough-textured "Gant de Massage", or massage glove. It comes in a variety of fabrics from wool to vegetable fibre.

In this country, a specialty bath shop or the bath department of a larger store can supply the item. However, a moderately-firm, natural bristled brush could well serve in the same capacity. Or one could grow the old-fashioned dishcloth gourds. From these, when they are dried, the extracted inner sponge becomes the massage glove that sloughs off dead skin and prepares one for sleep.

To eliminate the need for sleeping pills which bring unfortunate side effects with their repose, calcium could well be called the wise man's tranquilizer. Nerve-endings in the healthy body are coated with calcium. This produces the peaceful state which eliminates vague irritations. When calcium is lacking the body's need for this mineral is made known by constant waves of distress calls which produces the jitteryness we call "nerves", which in turn prevents sleep.

According to nutritionist Adelle Davis, two grams of calcium a day are required to overcome insomnia. But the problem today is how to get this quantity with our devitalized foods. An effort should be made to include in the diet sturdy-leafed vegetables and sunflower and sesame seeds—all high in calcium.

The Headstand can be practiced to great benefit by those who have trouble falling asleep. Simply arise and go into this position near your bed. After a few minutes in this inverted pose, sleep usually comes quite swiftly once you return to bed.

Some students have found the Swan to be even more helpful in bringing sleep than the Headstand. One woman discovered that on nights when sleep was elusive, she was able to fall asleep within minutes of going into the third position of the Swan. This is the position where the thighs are pressing against the abdomen and the head is inclined downward.

For others, completing the Swan exercise several times very slowly brings complete body relaxation. There is no doubt that the relaxed position of the Swan offers complete abandon and peace.

Foods To Be Avoided By Insomniacs

Usually it is wise to avoid any coffee or tea in the evening hours, unless they are of the herb or grain variety. Spicy dishes and heavy meals are another deterrent to sound sleep. Try to take most of your liquids during the daytime hours, rather than in the evening. Do not read or watch anything of an excitable nature that will arouse emotions late in the day.

CHAPTER SIXTEEN - MENTAL ATTITUDE MAKES THE DIFFERENCE

The dissatisfaction that is rife in so many lives seems to be increasing daily. What is it that sets the lines of annoyance in a pretty woman's face and places a perpetual scowl on a man's face? While these people may have much or little in the way of material wealth, the lines of dissatisfaction and annoyance are usually indicative of poverty in some area of greater importance than material possessions.

Somewhere along the pathway of mental and physical development a person can be detoured. Lacking some item considered necessary to creature comfort, perhaps a self-promise of success in this world is made. That first awareness of material lacking can change the charting of a life. The pursuit of sensual satisfaction can blot out fine motives for living, and a meaningful life can be lost in a drive to own more and more things and garner power.

It would seem that education as to the true values in life should commence very early. Those people who are the happiest, most beautiful, and contented, are not necessarily those who have amassed many tangible items of wealth. On the contrary, they are people who could be plucked up out of their present situation and placed in another, and instead of growing bitter or resentful, they would meet the new situation as they had met others—with a positive, constructive approach.

The wealth of a contented mind is a priceless possession. Such a mind would seek out the more substantial rewards of a world wherein qualities of contentment are the real rewards, rather than mere material possessions.

While one would not want to be without certain creature comforts, in our society today there is far too much time spent on the acquisition of material wealth. This too often controls the drives and yearnings of the inner man.

Yoga believes that all true happiness, wealth, power, and health lie in respecting oneself enough to avoid the pitfalls of poor living habits which lead to useless living. In learning to appreciate oneself, one is led to bring out one's finest physical and mental qualities. The resultant good health will then free one to grow spiritually and turn to one's fellow man with sincere motives.

Liking Oneself

Before any problem can be solved in mathematics, certain values have to be known. One cannot determine the value of x until one knows what y represents. While quantities and absolutes may remain unknown, there must be present a certain factor of knowledge.

It is the same with an individual. In order to correct faults and strengthen areas, one must know what these faults are, and wherein a weakness might lie. Yoga believes that in order to rebuild a body, one must know the body and be able to ascertain its weaknesses and its strengths. Then and only then can a course of action for improvement commence. The same theory applies to mental problems. In order to bring about a desired change of mind and create a healthy and peaceful attitude, one must know in what areas one is vulnerable.

The belief of Yoga is that one should take a clear, unbiased look at oneself, taking into full account both good and bad traits.

It is only logical that one must face oneself as a stranger and look at oneself objectively in order to draw up a proper list of corrective actions.

Make out an actual chart. Create a complete dossier of physical characteristics with honesty as the guiding factor. Describe your body as you honestly see it. Arrange in detail the qualities missing and the qualities desired. Face the problem head-on and sweep all doubt from the mind. If the body is large, small, flabby, or ill-formed, accept this as physical appearance that can, if desired, be changed to some degree.

After completing this detailed chart, begin on the mental. Name attitudes, traits, and habits. If you are subject to cynicism, irritability, boredom, or wrath, write them down.

Now, aim for the rational ideal. Remember to be realistic. If one's nature is to be retiring, it is hardly reasonable to decide that one should become an extrovert. Instead, aim for what is comfortably practical for you as an individual. Sometimes it is necessary merely to chip away at self-consciousness that perhaps creates or contributes to the retiring attitude, in order to bring one in closer contact to others.

In such a case, one might learn to listen while another speaks, in order to forget one's own preoccupation with oneself. One can reach out and help someone else as another means of forgetting self.

Yoga believes that only in knowing and appreciating oneself can one move beyond a constant petty self-involvement. As long as there is a pain or an ache in the body or mind, there will be a distraction, and a limited ability to move on to more worthwhile occupations than self-concern.

It is for this reason that Yoga suggests one get to know oneself. In that way, all discordant notes can be corrected, and the path to greater freedom and accomplishment achieved. Certainly a musician cannot perform to the best of his ability if he has an ache between the shoulders. Nor can a woman achieve her goal of complete femininity if she is bulging at the waistline or stricken with frequent headaches.

Yoga says that in order to make progress with ourselves we must first of all like ourselves. This is not an easy accomplishment for those in the Western world. One is taught from the earliest years not to think of oneself, as this is considered selfish. But there is a tremendous difference between self-discovery and mere egotism.

A genuine concern for onself has nothing to do with self-preoccupation. The one brings the body and mind to its top level of performance, the other is mentally crippling.

All the teachings of Yoga are based on the art of self-discipline. But if one does not like oneself, it is not possible to practice this art. As an example, when one goes to a doctor for help in an area of health, and the doctor says one must stop smoking, though the patient may actually desire to quit, it is not possible to do so merely because the doctor recommends it.

Only if the patient cares enough for his own life will he be concerned with his condition. Only then can he rid himself of this habit, or eliminate any other deleterious practice. His fears may be intense, yet if he cares more for the destructive pleasure of smoking than he cares for his body's health, he will follow the dictates of his compulsion rather than the concerned advice of his physician.

An effective method of self-improvement that will help to remove habits which create self-dislike is also a very simple one. Each day sit for a few minutes and think about some aspect of the personality or personal self. Take one thing at a time and try to change it for the better.

For some, this is an easier approach to self-betterment than the fully drawn up list of unfavorable characteristics one seeks to change. Again, one must choose that path that will best lead to his own goal.

If there is a tendency to be short of temper, work on patience and understanding. If the bad habit is one of interruption when another is speaking, learn to hold your voice and listen. You will grow richer by your silence.

This is not an easy lesson to learn, nor is it easy to put into practice. Its simplicity must be weighed against our own entrenched ideas of value and self-importance. But the goal is important enough to make the effort worthwhile. For if we can change our meaner habits, we learn to appreciate ourselves. And if one has real concern for oneself, one can then help others, for one is released from the time-consuming passions of envy, resentfullness, and bitterness that cut us off from our fellow men.

Physical Tension

Tension in the average body today is an almost unbelievable force of deterioration. This is especially true here in the western hemisphere. As our way of living spreads out over the world, our varieties of illness seem to accompany it. Mania for a certain standard of living, which we are convinced is a blueprint for day-to-day survival, demands ever more possessions and artificial means of amusement. And with this passion for acquiring another car, a larger home, a swimming pool or boat, individual tensions assume even larger proportions.

There is a drive to succeed, to acquire, and to participate in more ways than the average body can handle without eventually breaking down. The slow, measured tempo of living has now been relegated to "vacation time." During this brief period ranging from a week to perhaps a month, the average American hopes to unwind from a year's accumulation of stress and strain.

Psychologists say this cannot be done successfully; that relaxation should be on a continual basis. Even if accumulated tensions could be drained away, like removing diseased blood, and a transfusion of serenity restored to the body, this once yearly rest and relaxation could not prevent one from succumbing to renewed assaults throughout the following year.

In addition to our own problems, we are faced with a multitude of world problems with which we concern ourselves, and most of them seem unsolvable. Because of this, we cannot sleep, we overeat, and as a result we become nervous, jittery and over-weight.

The first step toward a solution of our ills would be to differentiate between physical and mental tensions. Though they are related, we must think of them separately in order to overcome them.

Physically, we are an underactive nation. We do not use our bodies as we should and we build ill upon ill, never really strengthening our bodies to sustain us in a demanding world. Each year another labor-saving device deprives the body of an opportunity for honest exercise.

It is no longer as fashionable to walk as it once was. Families go for drives along crowded, littered highways instead of going for long, peaceful walks. Lawns are mowed by riding atop an efficient little machine, and thus enforced exercise is gone. Engine-powered boats skim over lakes and rush one up and down a river or bay like a dragonfly skimming over surface water. But a dragonfly propels himself, and profits from the movement. There is little exercise benefit from riding in a boat.

Rowing or paddling down a peaceful stream is a lost art. Gardens are roto-tilled, and rug-beating wands are antique collectors' items. We have become a nation of sedentary people.

Progress has given us a softer, easier life. Yet our national health is dipping below that of other civilized countries who have not advanced so rapidly, technologically, as we. The life expectancy of Americans has not increased since 1955, and the latest figures indicate it may be falling slightly.

Almost any form of physical movement is relaxing, if done with proper consideration for the body. Another means of relieving physical tension is to talk to the body. During isolated moments of the day, study yourself and your attitudes. See if you can find an area of tenseness in the body. Check for tight muscles and then talk to the body and instruct it to relax.

This practice invariably will bring you greater ease, and along with an increase in energy, will help you to function better during the day and to sleep better at night.

Mental Tension

Hatha Yoga teaches that you cannot successfully soothe the mind and raise it to its highest level of performance until you have acknowledged the ills of the body and corrected them. It is for this reason that we work first on taking the physical body through planned movements and exercises before we begin to expect improvement in the mind. But at the same time, the mind must be disciplined and aided, no less than the body.

While it is natural to be concerned about our various problems in life, most of us spend a great amount of time worrying in a negative way. Let's examine this habit.

Much of our worry is done in anticipation. We pose a hypothetical "What will I do if..." and in the majority of cases this problem will never arise. This means we have spent time arousing our distress for no valid reason. In other words, we worry unnecessarily. Then by the time we do have a legitimate concern, we are so tense and emotional that we are in no condition to take the right action to solve the problem.

Yoga says we should remove unnecessary worry from our minds. In this way, we will be more relaxed and capable of solving real problems.

Breathing Control

When we become distressed, our breathing usually becomes heavy and fast, our blood pressure rises, the heartbeats come at a faster rate, and shortly, we are losing control of ourselves. In order to avoid this, we must establish control over our breathing at the moment that worry commences.

We can accomplish this by taking slow, deep breaths. Though our anxiety may remain in spite of the deep breathing, we will be able to control the emotion, and thereby deal more effectively with the problem that produced this situation.

An excellent illustration of this occurred recently when a young woman alone in her apartment awakened to find two intruders in her bedroom. Their voices, discussing the harm they planned to her, had aroused her from sleep. Though she knew instant terror as she looked up at them from her vulnerable position, this disciplined young woman managed to hold onto her control.

"What do you think you are doing in here?" she shouted at them, jumping from the bed as she did so and springing to stand before an opened window.

Confronted with this positive defense, the housebreakers paused only a moment, then raced down the stairs, leaving the young woman shaking from her experience, but unharmed.

It is in this manner that mental discipline will come to the aid of the body every time. If the woman had succumbed to terror, had allowed her fright to interfere with her breathing to the point that she could not raise her voice above a whisper (as is frequently the case when fear takes control), then her weakness could have added impetus to the intruders' thoughts of violence.

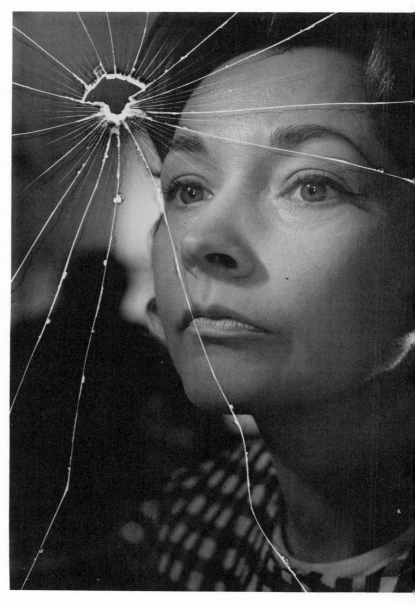

MENTAL ATTITUDE MAKES THE DIFFERENCE

Another devastating emotion is that of anger. Many of us in this nation are angry people. The tempo of our lives is not conducive to much harmony. Because of the smoldering anger which one sees and experiences daily in relationships with others, our bodies are poised for battle much of the time. We have to find peaceful sanctuaries in our private lives in order to regain our composure.

Sadly enough, much of this hostility and preparation for battle begins in our closest family relationships. But it can also arise from business contracts or such impersonal situations as making a simple purchase in a shop. Because of the prevalence of anger within us, only a minor incident is needed to cause a flareup that involves the entire body in this destructive action.

In a large family, with all members preparing for the day ahead, these conflicts can become a major upheaval, bringing blinding rage to those involved. In this manner, a chaotic episode leaves the injured party brooding all day over insults, real or imagined, and possible "revenge".

One mother of three boys said she was always exhausted by 8:30 A.M., when the last of her children finally left for school. The two older ones managed to get themselves under way with only minor conflicts. But the youngest son would often feign sickness to avoid going to school.

"No matter how much preparation I make the night before for a smooth morning departure," she said, "Bobby always managed to lose something at the last minute, develop an imagined sore throat, or just flatly state he didn't feel like catching the bus."

Her response was to scurry around searching for the lost object while scolding Bobby soundly for his lack of cooperation, or to accuse him of wading in the creek deliberately the day before, or, when he was the most obstinate, simply threatening to take away privileges should he fail to catch the bus.

She learned to change her tactics.

"Of course you may stay home," she informed her son who was already tensed for battle. She patted his head and said, "Your poor dear. You may stay home and help mommy clean house the way you did when you were a little boy."

Bobby stared at his mother, the rebellion gone from his eyes. "Bobby no longer does battle with me since he found I am not an enemy," the happy woman related.

There had been something in the mother's morning attitude of desperation that Bobby sensed, and to which he responded in kind. Anger begets anger, and it wasn't until the mother realized her own tense preparation for fury that she was able to discipline herself into the role of an agreeable person—able to help her children, rather than shove them into their day.

If we take time to realize that tension has a great deal to do with our hasty anger, we will be in a better position to deal with it. Hostility, resentment, annoyance, and scorn should never be aimed at another. Since these expressions are usually a part of our daily lives, it is not easy to dispose of them. But Yoga suggests policing ourselves in an effort to rid ourselves of these useless emotions. It is by this method of discipline that we can eliminate tensions, thereby benefitting ourselves and others.

Knowledge

The study and practice of Yoga teaches us that each day should be a time of learning and correcting. Yoga says we should always be ready to benefit from life itself. Aside from taking in new knowledge every day, we should also never repeat a mistake. For each new day gives us a chance to correct old errors. This is our way of profiting from past mistakes instead of "chalking" anything up as a total loss.

An indifferent attitude about a mistake means one has gained nothing from experience. To remain at one level of performance all one's life would be dull indeed. One should be able to meet new challenges and advance both spiritually and mentally. If there is a listless attitude toward life, then one's days become as stagnant as a small pond that has no source and no outlet.

We all know people who never seem to advance in anything they do. We also know people whose speech remains undeveloped and whose thoughts never have the freshness of new ideas, or new exposures.

These are people who have not matured in spite of their years. They are people who have not learned to profit from past mistakes or to go on to a higher level of performance, whether in the home, at work, or in a relationship with other people.

Yoga says we must take the time to analyze objectively what we have been exposed to, and what we have learned each day. Above all, we must keep our minds open. It is in this manner one achieves prosperity and peace. Observing and understanding the world around one brings about a closer relationship between oneself and others, and this in turn brings peace and removes a feeling of inadequacy.

There should never come a period in our lives when we decide we have acquired all of the knowledge we need. Or that any additional knowledge would be of no value to us. As long as we can expand our knowledge, our minds will continue to grow. And growth is life itself.

Mental Attitudes As Reflections

Just as temporary joy will momentarily paint radiance across a face and reflect a flashing happiness, so too will more permanent emotions etch a face with lines that indicate one's outlook on life. It is not for nothing that in depictions of drama, classic masks of comedy and tragedy are represented by upturned and downturned mouth positions. The lines on the face are a mirror to the personality that lies beneath.

MENTAL ATTITUDE MAKES THE DIFFERENCE

A sincerely pleasant, outgoing person often has a look of roundness on the cheeks whereas a bitter, unhappy person shows descending lines that resemble little exclamation points of disaster. This is not by chance. The happier person uses his facial muscles in expressing pleasure. Therefore his face is more firm and consequently, less aged in appearance than the person who allows his depressed mental attitude to set downward lines into the facial areas.

The upward lift of the face as it forms a smile is a potent exercise against aging. Not only is one profiting from the rewards of a smile, but the pleasure is reflected on another's face in response.

Positive emotions such as joy, pleasure, delight, happiness, and contentment—when reflected on the face—tell a brief story of what one is experiencing inwardly. And there is no successful way to conceal what one is experiencing. One can outwardly cover up a moment of awkwardness or displeasure. But the lines do get etched when they reflect a daily attitude. Since one who experiences frequent or constant displeasure usually does not make an attempt to conceal it, this emotion becomes embedded in lines and furrows and tautly-held lips, chin, or forehead.

There are other ways that mental attitudes write a story across the face. The harried individual who drives himself to a point of exhaustion, like a keen bloodhound on the trail of some choice tidbit, develops the same vertical lines on the forehead as does the animal his behavior mimics.

A suspicious nature narrows the eyes and lessens their brilliance. The constricture of this area shortens the natural blood flow needed for clear vision. Instead of being receptive to explanation, the distrusting person constricts his mind even as he narrows his eyes.

Flittering, wavering eyes suggest an instability that will not permit composure. Serenity opens eyes wide to all around, and lends a steady gaze when another is speaking.

Clinging to sadness in one's life stunts development. Loss of a loved one is a difficult thing to accept, but there must be a higher belief that sustains one. Sorrow that cannot be changed should not be permitted to darken one's days indefinitely. Remembered deeds of kindness and love are a powerful light against the darkness of despair. Though darkness in itself may seem all enveloping, it has no real power. Light one candle and the blackness is swept away. We should live at all times in such a manner that one's relationship with others brings just such a brightness to mind.

Overcoming Negative Attitudes

One can overcome negative attitudes that spoil living in three ways. First, the physical condition must be improved. Second, one must learn to relax. Third, one must learn to employ persistent mental exercises that lift one out of the pettiness of thought that leads to this situation.

When the body is exercised daily and the glands are working properly, then nerves begin to relax. At this point, it is natural to become optimistic and philosophical. One then learns to take life as it comes, and to appreciate the very act of being alive. Triumphs come when one is able to turn the things around him into positive assets through the development of the mind.

Drugs

Yoga tells us that one should help oneself when ill, by correcting one's diet and by exercising one's body. In order to help effect a cure for a specific ailment, Yogis have used herbs, roots, and other natural growth from the earth. Here in the western part of the world, we use far too many drugs. If we have a headache, we automatically reach for an aspirin bottle. We don't question deeply enough what is causing the pain.

All around us, we are assaulted by news media and displays suggesting we buy different types of drugs for various ailments. These daily commands suggest that if we swallow a pill, we will be benefiting our bodies. But the contrary is true. One should be extremely careful about any medication one buys because of the persuasion of an advertisement.

So-called mind-expanding drugs are really mind-stultifying. No mind can be improved or function at its best when it is controlled by a drug.

The torpor which spreads over the body when the mind has been influenced by a drug may suggest to some that this is a form of release. But on the contrary, the body and mind are both imprisoned when drugs are used.

Euphoria of mind and body are obtainable through Yoga exercises and good nutrition alone, without any mechanical or artificial devices. There are those who are self-indulgent and do not care to take the time necessary to lead the body to this contented state. For them, drugs appear to be a short cut to Nirvana, or that perfect state of being. Actually, the narcotics used today are a short-cut to debilitation and death.

Yoga has successfully been used among groups of teenagers as a means of turning them away from drug taking. Such programs catch at these vulnerable youngsters and teach them the pleasure of good health stemming from a beautifully kept body. Once the student is introduced to the stimulation of deep breathing and the good effects of planned exercise, his inclination toward narcotics is usually removed.

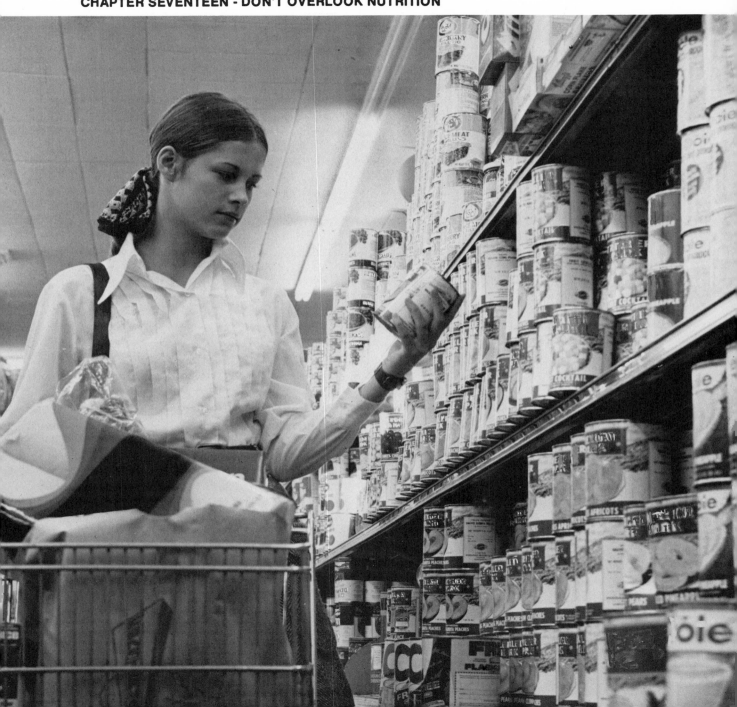

Who are the really beautiful people in the world? Jet-setters who have the means to order any and all of life that can be purchased, or the simply-living person who awakens with the sun and takes his sustenance from the living plants around him?

Because the peasant is living with true beauty if he has access to freshly grown food, that same food will help to make him a beautiful person. Beauty, then, is not so much in the eyes of the beholder as in the hands of the harvester.

Beauty does not come in pre-packaged containers, nor can it be poured from a can, thawed from a block of ice, or revitalized from a dehydrated form by adding water. Beauty is always original and unspoiled, as close to nature, and therefore as natural, as possible.

Food that is both beautiful and good is unspoiled, and changed as little as possible from its original condition. A field of growing grain is beautiful, a garden of green vegetables exquisite, and a tree filled with developing fruit a joy to the eyes. This is beauty growing and it is impossible to improve upon it. If we recognize beauty in its true form, as with growing things, and realize the fact that beauty can bestow beauty, then perhaps we should create a list of pure foods and change our present diet to include them all. Then we could profit from this formula for real and lasting beauty.

The world is hearing more and more about a group of people who live in the Himalayas—a good distance away—uncontaminated by civilization and basking in beauty, good health, and longevity. Their foods are simple and unprocessed. They harvest their vegetables from the fields and consume only fresh, untreated meats. Their grain is threshed and ground as they require it.

There are no canning plants, no frozen food industries, and no hot dog, hamburger, or soft-drink stands in their pristine country.

As our bewildered civilization in the West, which has come so far technically, tries to pull itself from the mire it has created, we look to the Hunzas in the Himalayas and know a sense of envy for their beautiful, uncomplicated, and unprocessed way of life.

The beliefs of Yoga are closely allied to the philosophy as lived by the Hunzas. Though the Hunzas are meat eaters in moderation, Yogis are vegetarians. But their reason for eliminating meat from their diet is based on a spiritual belief. This is their practice, and a custom of long standing. But since we in the Western world have not shared the same philosophical train of thought that would bring us to this conclusion, it is entirely appropriate for us to pursue our own customs regarding the consumption of meat, even as we derive infinite benefits from the Westernized version of this discipline.

Yoga believes that all food that we consume should be in a natural state. Since most of our foods are either preserved or treated otherwise with chemicals, this is difficult for us to achieve. However, with an understanding of what is taking place in the food industry, and with a general knowledge of the harmful additives placed in food to insure a long shelf life, we can learn to choose less damaging products and safeguard our health to a greater degree.

Purchasing wholesome, preservative-free food in America has become a time-consuming activity. When I lived in France and had American visitors, I would take them marketing with me to see the colorful stalls of crisp vegetables, picked that same morning in the countryside for the Paris markets. Marketing was an activity that required from one to two hours.

France has few supermarkets. Instead, one shop handles meats, another fish, another vegetables and fruits, another bread, another dairy products, and so on. Invariably, my friends would complain, "How can you stand this daily marketing in all these shops? I'd go out of my mind if I couldn't make all my purchases in one supermarket."

Now I am back in the States, and I find that in order to get unpreserved and reasonably fresh foods, I am spending from one to three hours a day driving miles to the roadside stand that has organically grown vegetables, to the farmer who sells raw milk, to the shop that sells fresh meat from animals that haven't been fattened with stilbestrol. Yet another source must be visited for unsprayed grains; and another for raw honey.

Meal planning by the homemaker today requires constant vigilance. If she is concerned with her health and that of her family, she must learn to read labels in order to avoid the multitude of additives placed in food. She must also examine produce for indications of poisonous sprays, and learn to pick and choose a few items in a wasteland of processed and adulterated food products. One can no longer buy a bag of apples and be assured of getting a simple food item. Many apples are waxed in order to insure a long shelf life. This is done even though the wax cannot be removed from the apple by any simple means, and even though wax is known to be carcinogenic.

Citrus fruits are pulled unripened from their branches without their full complement of vitamin C. They are then colored artificially for selling appeal, and passed on to an unsuspecting public.

Sweet potatoes and yams are now dyed red to achieve the same color the minerals in the soil used to give them. And whereas the red skins created by the rich minerals were delicious and healthful, the same cannot be said for the artificially dyed ones.

Acorn squash and rutabagas are dipped in paraffin. Cheeses are produced by chemical processing. Milk is heated to a high temperature which destroys the enzyme values, and then various synthetic vitamins are stirred in.

One can walk down the aisles of any supermarket in the country and try almost without success to find a pure and untreated food. The items offered for human consumption are artificially colored, frozen, exploded, dehydrated, fried, whipped, diluted, concentrated, refined, and degerminated.

And yet this country produces more food per capita than any other in the world. Our erroneous methods of getting the vast tonnage of food to the public are bringing about an increase in degenerative diseases that has placed us in the role of poorly fed people.

The popular picture of the rose-cheeked Gibson Girl beauty and the outdoor look of the handsome All-American boy doesn't really hold up today. No longer are we a nation of comfortable, well-built, and easily functioning people. Our institutions, both penal and mental, are filled with inmates suffering from nutritional deficiencies.

Our offices are staffed by nervous, ulcerous people. Homes are being torn apart by neurotic compulsions. Schools are filled with angry, insecure, and belligerent youngsters. Wherever one turns, one encounters hostility, annoyance, rejection, or brutality. Some attribute this to the rapidly increasing population. But many people in other societies have lived at close quarters without experiencing the instant anger one encounters today.

Youngsters in their teens and twenties seem the most susceptible to this breakdown of society. Coincidentally, it is they who are the most drawn to the non-nutritional diet; hamburgers, hot dogs, soft drinks, and potato chips have been the mainstays of their diet for most of the years of their lives.

Some attribute the present national distress to a new social awareness on the part of young people today. They say it is this that creates the rage that vandalizes and destroys private and public property and disrupts education across the country.

More likely, the constant anger and turmoil of our country can be laid at the door of nutritional deficiencies. When an animal is deprived of a suitable diet, he will develop a rage so intense that he will actually bite the hand that feeds him. Doesn't this same rule of nutrition apply to man?

If a human being is without the proper nutrients necessary for orderly function of both body and mind, it is not too far-fetched to imagine a similar reaction.

No one diet would be suitable for all, perhaps. In Yoga we teach that no two bodies are alike; that one cannot fairly compare one's body to another. The same applies to the practices of good nutrition. One must choose of all available foods those which bring the nutrients one's own body requires.

However, regardless of whether you are overweight, underweight, or both in different spots, for the next 6 weeks apply these basics:

—Eat no sugar whatsoever. It will take only two or three days to lose the desire for it.

—Eat at least one egg a day.

—Reduce or eliminate your consumption of bread. If you cannot give it up completely eat a coarse, whole grain bread and no more than two slices.

—Eat a high-protein food at every meal, including breakfast. Organ meats like liver, heart, kidneys, are particularly good. Use lean meats like turkey and round steak. Fish is fine. But no shellfish.

—Try to find a source of organically grown vegetables—health food stores frequently carry them. Don't stint on eating them. Eat a big salad every day and you can eat potatoes, too, baked or boiled rather than fried. Sweet potatoes are excellent. Dress your salads with a vegetable oil (sunflower, soy, corn) and apple cider vinegar. Garlic or raw onion will improve the flavor. Use raw fruits for desserts.

—Snack on nothing but raw seeds and nuts (sunflower seeds, walnuts, Brazil nuts and filberts taste good raw) or nuts that have been roasted in the shell.

—Take daily natural food supplements: fish liver oil for vitamins A and D, rose hips tablets for vitamin C, vitamin E capsules, brewer's yeast for B complex, bone meal and dolomite for minerals.

Vitamin intake is extremely important to the overall health and beauty of the body. While the right amounts of natural food many times insure the correct intake of needed nutrients, sometimes it is necessary to supplement a diet with extra vitamins. In fact, usually the appearance of the skin itself will give its own clues as to what is deficient for you in seemingly complete meals.

Lack of vitamin A in the diet soon shows itself in dryness, scaliness of the skin, and an aged look that can be corrected when this vitamin is increased.

Sources of this vitamin that is worth its weight in gold are fresh fruits, liver, fish, carrots, eggs, spinach, corn, fresh peas, green beans, and cucumbers, among others.

The absence of vitamin A within the body can stem from more than poor nutrition, though. Sometimes there is an inability within the body itself to utilize or store the proper amounts of specific vitamins. Defective intestinal absorption may produce severe effects that manifest themselves on the skin. In such cases, an increase in your intake of vitamin E will often facilitate vitamin A absorption. Medically administered therapeutic doses of vitamin A can bring about definite improvement in such skin conditions.

While some nutritionists feel one cannot take too many vitamins, especially if they are from natural sources, other research suggests that of all vitamins, A and D can be taken in quantities greater than needed by the body, and produce unwanted results. The Council on Foods and Nutrition says prolonged ingestion of A in excess of 50,000 USP units daily could be harmful. Toxicity usually disappears when dosage is discontinued.

One way to avoid this concern would be external application of vitamin A for skin eruptions due to its lack. This has proved extremely beneficial to persons suffering from a disorder in which the skin becomes sandpapery, and fine cracks appear around the ear, sometimes so deeply the fissures bleed. Daily applications of vitamin A in cream form are extremely helpful here. Vitamin A and D ointments, made from deodorized cod liver oil and possessing a pleasant texture and odor are readily available. There are also natural cosmetic creams enriched with vitamin A.

As for those nutritionists who say if one eats sensibly, he does not have to take additional vitamin supplements, the statement is no doubt made on the assumption that it is always possible to obtain fresh ripe food in the average market. Any housewife knows better. When vegetables are trucked in from distant parts of the country in the wintertime, days can elapse before they reach their final destination. Add several more days while they lie in their market places and you may have a total time lapse of nearly a week from the harvesting hour to the moment they are served on the table. Even more unfortunate, it has become a common practice to harvest unripe food, store it for months, and distribute it out of season for a higher price.

During this time, many vitamin losses are taking place within the now not-so-fresh food. Long exposure to air brings about the destruction of vitamin A. Dehydration also increases its deterioration. Is this food in its finest form? Are these wilted vegetables as full of nutrition as they started out? If not, then the suggestion that one does not need various supplements is not valid.

With the above loss, add to that the waste in food preparation. Since vitamin A is not water soluble, there is supposed to be no measurable loss here, but a long cooking process does its damage in destroying the vitamin. By the time the food is finally consumed, then, much of the value is gone and it becomes bulk, without the nutrition it started out with.

All this would seem enough reason to supplement the diet with added vitamins to insure even the basic requirements. For many years doctors have been treating serious acne cases with vitamin A. But how much better if nutrition were used as a preventive rather than a remedial action. It can certainly be done if you search for the right nutrition.

Always keep in mind the phrase "balanced nutrition" and its importance. Do not think that you can substitute for all else with one type food required for a specific part of a well functioning body and ignore the body's other needs. It is not one magical food but overall diet that leads to beauty. Examine your diet carefully, with pen and paper. Start with breakfast and write down everything you consume in the course of a day. Every sip and bite must be recorded.

Now try to determine accurately what proportion of your diet is protein, how much is refined starches and sugar and saturated fats, and how much is unheated, unsaturated vegetable oil. Lumping together the refined starches, sugars and solid fats like butter or canned cooking fats, because they are all equally bad for health and beauty, will give you a new viewpoint on whether or not your diet is balanced. You may well find that the single category of health-wrecking foods far outbalances the other two.

Figure out this total at the end of the day, or try it over several days for better results, but total your intake at the end of each day. After you have the results, then examine the overall picture and see what changes for the better you should make. You may be surprised to find the degree to which you're actually starving your body of needed high grade proteins, a category that includes only eggs, meat and fish. Most of us can always cut down on sugar, wheat flour and fat. That means elimination or sharp reduction of bread, pastries, cakes, many pork products, ground meat that has been puffed out with fat, and even soups that have not had the fat skimmed from the top, if prepared with meat. We do it by increasing the intake of eggs, lean meat, complex carbohydrates such as fruit and vegetables, and seed foods like nuts, wheat germ, sunflower seeds.

Learning to practice good nutrition is far less complicated than having to cope with the ills of a body lacking the food it needs. By feeding the body natural, unadulterated nutrients, one can avoid many hours spent in a doctor's waiting room, hospital stays, and time lost from work. By following a natural food diet, one develops boundless energy, builds a foundation of good health, and creates a beautifully functioning mind and body.

Grains in a natural state play an important role in a Yoga diet. This immediately rules out the bleached white flour almost universally sold in the markets. Unbleached flour is little better. In the refining process, the germ and the outer layers have been removed, even though it is here that the most vital substances are found.

Wheat germ is removed from flour during the milling process because it is highly perishable. The oils in the germ grow rancid very quickly and thereby limit the shelf life of the milled flour. In order to produce a food staple that can sit for many months in a shop without showing signs of age, all the life is removed from the product, and the inert powder is sold to the unwary buyer.

A tragic example of the harmfulness that comes from using white flour, or any of its products, lies in the story of a hunter marooned in an isolated cabin in Canada during a long siege of snowstorms. For a month of enforced isolation, the hunter had only white flour and tea from which to prepare his meals.

His diary is a day-by-day account of his failing health as he continued to bake bread from the white flour which was his only food source. Finally, after detailing the suffering of swollen limbs, rotting gums, and eventual complete immobility, he died of scurvy.

There was still a large container of flour found in the cabin with the hunter who died from this strange form of starvation. The vitamin and mineral deficiency of the flour brought on scurvy which caused death. The hunter would have done far better, had he known, to scrape the bark off the trees and to dig for a few roots under the snow.

Why would anyone, recognizing the harmful effects of white flour as evidenced by this story, choose to continue to eat a food that not only is lifeless, but life-draining as well?

Had the flour been left in its original state, the hunter could have gotten through his ordeal alive.

White sugar is another refined, nutritionless food to be avoided. This processed product leads to dental decay, removes the vitamin B from the body and upsets the blood sugar level, among other destructive acts. If left in its raw state, sugar at least supplies minerals, removed during the refining process.

White rice is yet another example of a devitalized food that is passed off as a good food staple. The polishing process used to remove the outer covering also destroys the B vitamins and produces a lifeless food of no significant value. Again, here is a grain that is delicious and wholesome when eaten in its natural state. But during the milling process, a food capable of giving life is reduced to nutritionless bulk.

Though even in the Far East polished white rice is used almost to the exclusion of the natural brown rice, General Chiang Kai-shek, searching for a way to increase the energy of his troops, had the customary polished white rice replaced with brown rice, to the great benefit of his army.

The instant mixes of white, dehydrated rice marketed as convenience foods are so completely without taste and value as to be practically worthless. Such rice is dependent on hot or spicy sauces to restore any semblance of taste.

Honey is yet another food that is sold to the consumer considerably changed from its original raw state. Suppliers are permitted to heat honey up to 140 degrees Fahrenheit and still label it "uncooked". Yet, at 140 degrees, many of the enzymes are destroyed, thus lessening the value of honey as a food.

The heating is done in order to prevent crystallization of the honey. In large part, the public has asked for this. The average housewife is not eager to buy a jar of honey that looks partially solidified or granulated. She knows that the crystals prevent easy pouring. But does she know that for the sake of convenience, she is shortchanging herself and her family? It is a very simple matter to set a jar of crystallized honey in a pan of hot water and have it return to a liquid state within a short time. This is far better than having a food processor heat it to a temperature so high that desperately needed food enzymes are lost from the diet.

The list of tampered-with foods is long. It is enough to say: avoid any and all of these processed foods, and try to find a source that can supply you with food as nature intended it—fresh from the vine, the ground, or the animal, with as little interference as possible from man.

Food As A Health and Beauty Need

Complaints of bodily ills are increasing along with external complexion distresses that send women flocking to the cosmetics counter seeking a new cream or miracle coverup. Yet the cure for these ills can be found in a living food source. Dry skin becomes elastic and youthful when the diet is corrected and planned to include as many living foods as possible.

Lank and oily hair becomes thick and attractive when there is enough protein taken in. Since the hair is one of the first places to show that the body is being starved of needed nutrients, it is of the greatest importance to keep a close watch over this part of the body. Look to the diet if there is a feeling of lifelessness or trouble with the hair.

Wrinkles can be reduced and controlled, aches and pains that paint a look of age across the face can be lessened, and a host of other complaints can be righted with a sensible natural diet. Beauty of body can come about only through good nutrition and sufficient exercise and sleep. The outer appearance must be based on the intake of productive foods. In order to create, a substance must first be alive itself. Obviously, live foods are going to do a better job of creating or developing a healthy and beautiful body than devitalized, dead foods.

Yoga believes it is easy enough to find the guidelines to live foods as opposed to dead foods. Anything that has growing potential is of greater value than something that would decay if put in the ground to grow. A dried bean has more life to it than the sodden and soaked-in-sauce bean that comes from the can as a "baked bean". Plant the dried bean and from the power within the seed, germination commences and in a matter of days life is pushing out of the soil. No matter how old the dried bean is, it is still filled with life. Seeds that were placed in Egyptian tombs thousands of years ago have been planted and have produced healthy vines.

Food from growing plants, taken from the vine to the table so to speak, will supply the body far more effectively than will a dead food.

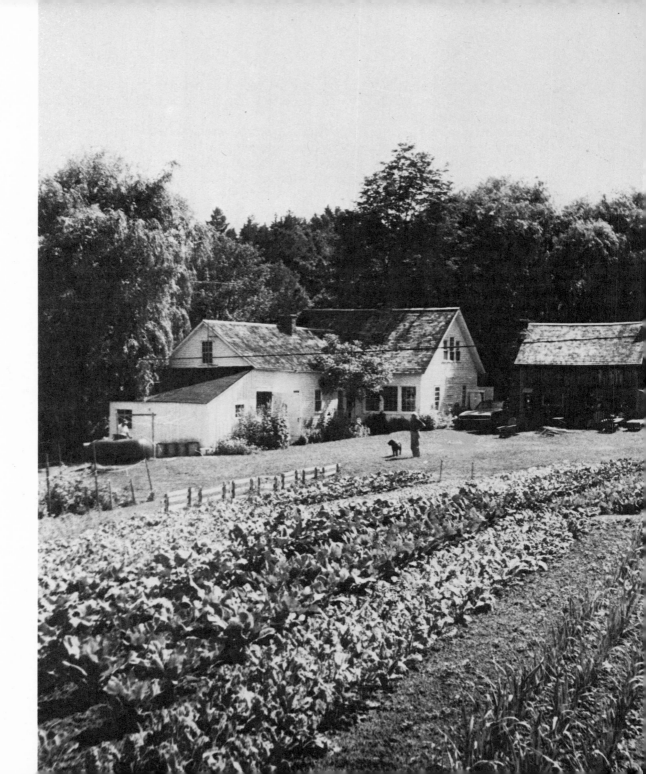

CHAPTER EIGHTEEN - "ORGANIC" IS A WAY OF LIFE

It would seem that if more time could be given to nutritional education and the implementing of laws to protect the public from harmful food products so lacking in nutrition, personal ills would not become social ills. There would be less need for funds to weigh the hazard of drug taking, to probe into the causes of the criminal mind, mental and physical diseases, and early deterioration and aging of the body. These things are all evidence that vital food values are lacking in our diet, and because of a growing concern, there is today a heartening trend back toward the nutritional values of yesterday.

A hunger of palatable "real" foods, as opposed to tasteless plastic non-foods, has been aroused. Co-ops, where the freshness of food can be better-guarded, are springing up around the country. A greater and more intense interest in organic farming has developed. People are beginning to become concerned about the death of our farmland, and the increase in debilitating diseases. Armed with statistics that show our national level of health to be dropping, and with an upward rise in cancer, heart disease, tuberculosis, arteriosclerosis, and arthritis, people are asking questions which the food industry refuses to answer.

The problem has been with us for so long and is of such huge proportions that one wonders if anything can be done about it. For with the landing of the first settlers on these shores a few hundred years ago, the first step on the path to our present starved soil was taken.

For a short while the new American farmers did listen to the ways of the Indian. These wise native husbandmen showed the newcomers how to enrich and fertilize the ground with fish caught from the lakes and seas. And how to use seaweed as a replenisher of minerals that were being taken from the soil with every crop.

When this practice was followed, the corn grew tall and rich, and the pumpkins were juicy and large. But the influx of pioneers was greater than the number of Indian instructors. And the farmer was mesmerized by the rich black loam from which a seed would spring without coaxing. He forgot all about the hard work that goes into caring for the soil.

He forgot the heavy loads of shells he had hauled from the oceanside and crushed and returned to the earth for their natural mineral value. Inland farmers forsook the hoarding and spreading of manures, so vital to provincial farmyards throughout Europe, where the soil remains rich and productive.

Here in the new land the farmer felt freed from this. So he blithely planted and reaped, believing the richness of the earth was everlasting and beyond abuse. For centuries the new land had grown forests and lush meadow grasses. And these in time had returned to the earth to add their own richness to the receptive soil. It was as though the new land had been composed of one large mulch pit.

So the uncaring farmer took crop after crop from a generous soil and never gave anything back. But as forests were cut down and the meadows disappeared, the replenishers of the soil went with them. As the soil grew poorer, the farmer gathered his family and moved on, extending his poor farming practices westward, southward and northward. He was always searching for the good land—the soil that needed only clearing and thrusting in of seeds to provide the needed food to feed the hardy generations of early Americans.

As he moved westward, the farmer further denuded the land and removed the life-giving properties from the soil. He cleared away forest and brush and wantonly destroyed the wildlife around him. The barrens of the Midwest show the rape of the land he left in his wake. The great dust storms of the 1930's were caused by the removal of all natural plant life by these unthinking land destroyers.

So the tradition was born of taking from the soil without replenishing. Some farmers did hold to the old ways of farming and replenishing the land. But these were usually the ones who remained in one area and they were few, for America was on the move.

Farms were larger here than they had been in the old country. In Europe, each farm family had perhaps a cow, some sheep, chickens, pigs and a horse or other work animal. Enough waste was collected from these animals to fertilize their small farms. But in the new land, with much more acreage under cultivation per family, a farmer could seldom put into the soil enough to compensate for what he took out.

In time, the chemical fertilizers which we rely upon today were developed. These inorganic stimulators are a poor substitute for the natural minerals that have long since disappeared from grounds under intensive commercial cultivation.

Now, with the growing national concern about our poor health, the swing back to organic farming is bringing its own rewards to those involved.

With organic methods, soil can be restored to its original richness. For intensely depleted areas, it may take as long as two or three years, but that is not really so long, considering how long it took to deteriorate to its present state.

Consider the case of one young man who managed to buy a small development home for his family, with a moderate sized lot. Not only does he grow enough vegetables and fruits to feed his family for many months of the year, but the food is produced from soil that has been completely reclaimed and is as rich as organic farming can make it.

This surburban farmer puts everything he can find of an organic nature into his compost pile in order to break it down and eventually return the results to the soil. Even old leather shoes find their way into the rich compost heap. Every shred of kitchen refuse is turned back into rich, black soil. He regularly visits nearby stables for manure to enrich his garden. He haunts the fish markets and cheerfully carries off the fish heads, entrails, and bones. In time, this will decompose into the rich humus that produces food for beauty and health.

Organic farming is not only a means of reclaiming one's health, it is actually a great and rewarding challenge. Also, once the need for this way of life is recognized, it helps to bring a family closer together. For Americans have always drawn together in times of great need.

And surely, there is no need greater than that of reducing the sickness that is blanketing our country as a result of improper nutrition.

Good nutrition, then, is not only knowing how to choose a well-balanced diet that will keep a family free of illness; it is also a recognition of the values that go into the food itself. It is the act of locating a source of organically grown food, or cultivating it oneself.

Only the poultry farmer who permits his chickens to peck unpenned about the yard, enabling them to have a diet rich in minerals, can sell you fertilized eggs that help build healthy skin and hair. The imprisoned fowl that live out their lives in electrically controlled plants, never receiving the beneficial effects of sunshine or minerals from the earth, cannot hope to produce an egg with yolk the color of sunlight.

Good nutrition is gathering the youngest dandelion leaves, rich in potassium and calcium, as they push upward from the lawn, and chopping them raw into a salad with other fresh, untreated vegetables and herbs.

It is the knowledge that parsley should be consumed and not used only as a decoration to please the eye. The vitamin A in it will do much for the eyes, and its iron content will purify the blood.

Good nutrition is planting fruit trees in place of ornamental trees, if ground space is limited. One or two fruit trees will boost a family's health by providing a naturally rich source of vitamins.

There are countless ways to improve the health of your family and to wage a personal battle against the dead foods that lie so limply in the vegetable bins of shops across the country. Such a plan requires thought and some work in the implementation. But the rewards are an increase in energy, beauty, and a more active role in life.

Raw sunflower seeds head the list of beauty foods for the entire family. One sees the people in the Soviet Union walking down the street or sitting in the parks cracking the little seeds in order to extract the delicious nut-like kernels within the hulls. While an expert can manage this hull opening with agility, using both his tongue and teeth, it does require a certain expertise. Fortunately, already-hulled sunflower seeds are available at any health food store.

Instead of buying boxes of chocolates, spend your money on a bag of sunflower seeds, and place them invitingly next to a bowl of dates, figs, raisins, or other fresh or dried fruit. The rich nutrition of the sunflower seed can perhaps be explained by this plant's interesting ability to continually face the sunshine as it turns on its stalk throughout the day.

From early morning until the last rays disappear in the early evening, this flower of the sun pivots toward its source of life. As a result the seeds yield vitamin D and calcium for the natural serenity that creates beauty and helps to clear up skin outbreaks.

For those with a sweet tooth, good nutrition does not ban all confections, by any means. In fact, once you have been weaned away from harmful refined sugar products, guilt disappears when you reach for a nourishing and tasty fruit and nut candy. A mixture of dried fruits, honey, and nuts can be quickly prepared and kept at hand. A child brought up on this type of candy will be spared many hours in a dental chair. At the same time, these mixtures of unrefined foods are sources of good nutrition and of boundless energy.

Pumpkin seeds are another delicious between-meal snack that contributes to the healthful functioning of the inner organs.

Get rid of the spicy condiments that create a blotched complexion and replace them with simple herbs that add an exotic taste to any meal. A bowl of chives growing in the kitchen window, a bowl of watercress forming a miniature garden, a pot of parsley all provide a constant source of nutrition and flavor.

Good nutrition calls for a daily green vegetable in the diet. In order to get the most value from such a vegetable, one should pull it fresh from its stalk or vine and use it within minutes of its harvest. Since this is not always practical, we should look for alternate means of supplying the essentials for beauty.

For example, diets containing live food will supply the body with the materials required for restorative and maintenance work. One of the finest of all live foods is the sprout. No medicine can restore a lost complexion to its former beauty so quickly as a daily handful of raw sprouts. There is no cosmetic that can melt away blemishes so effectively as these rich, full-of-life green sprouts that hold within them the essentials for the beauty that we crave. Sprouts are a concentrated form of beauty food; only a handful a day will help to bring beauty to the body.

For those with only a small summer garden from which to choose their vegetables, and for those without a garden at all, the centuries old Oriental custom of growing sprouts from seed, to serve as fresh, green vegetables, is ideal. Sprouting brings a maximum of good benefits with a minimum of effort, cost, and space.

Seeds contain the greatest amount of protein of all vegetables, and their high vitamin and mineral content is increased as the seeds first begin their development into a growing plant. Until seeds are allowed to absorb a quantity of water, their tough, dehydrated form conceals the dormant life of a sleeping giant. Then, after adequate absorption of water, and with a suitably warm temperature, the life within the seed stirs, expands, and bursts forth with full regenerative power.

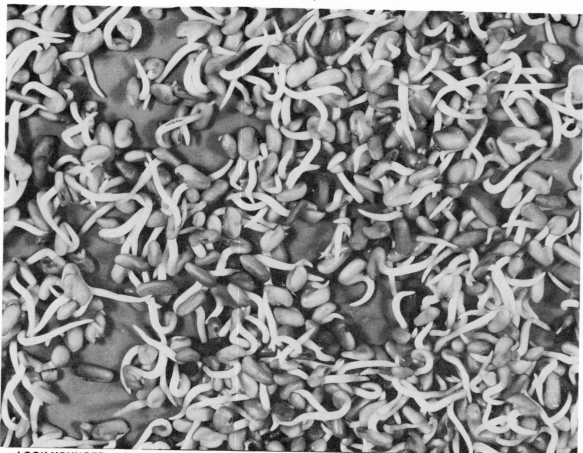

The unsprouted seed is truly akin to a sleeping beauty. Upon germination, the concentration of life within the small seed expands and multiplies to the point that eating the sprouting seed is like drinking from the fountain of youth.

It is this power of generation that, when included in the daily diet, will bring new life to the body and rejuvenate a tired and aging skin. The use of sprouts, grown from seeds, nuts, and grain, is one of the most rewarding of all nutritional practices. Glowing health will replace a wan complexion when one or more varieties of sprouts are consumed daily.

Easy to grow, these little plants require no soil, no sunlight, and little attention to produce a harvest of vitamins and minerals, designed to invigorate the starved complexion and tired body. All that is required is a handful of seeds, and either a pan or a glass jar with a wide opening.

Select the seed you would most enjoy. Among the seeds from which to choose, are mung beans, soybeans, and lentils. The grains include alfalfa, wheat, barley, and millet. Smaller seeds which produce a zesty salad type green are radish, fenugreek, and sunflower. For a quick, guaranteed crop, the mung bean seems to be the winner. But since the values of other seeds are high, they too should be used.

It is important that any seeds used for sprouting should not be treated with mercury or any other fungicide. To prepare the seeds for germination and growth, place a tablespoon of them in a glass of warm water and leave them to soak overnight. Place them in a strainer the following morning and rinse them in clear, lukewarm water. Try to sprinkle the seeds down the length of the jar, then place it on its side, leaving the mouth open. Keep the jar in a warm place out of drafts, in the kitchen or elsewhere. Water the seeds by a slight sprinkling every three or four hours, or as they require it. Do not place the seeds in the sunlight, at least not until their leaves have fully formed.

After one or two days, a tiny root will thrust forth. By the third or fourth day little leaves will appear, and it is then, when two leaves have opened, that the sprouts are at their richest in food value. Time required for sprouting varies from two to five days, dependent on the room temperature and the type of seed.

The food value of the sprout decreases steadily after this point. Gather the green plants, rinse them off and plan to use them immediately in a salad, to top a cup of soup, steamed with other vegetables, or to add to another raw or cooked vegetable. Nutritionally, they are of the greatest value when eaten raw, but some object to the earthy taste, which disappears with brief steaming of three or four minutes.

Another tasty use of sprouts is in sandwiches, fillings and omelets. Each time you consume even a handful of freshly grown sprouts, you can be confident of having used one of the richest and most nourishing foods available anywhere. Because of the miracle of their own growth, the benefits to both skin and body will seem a near miracle, too.

Types of Food

Some foods are more beneficial taken raw, but obviously, others are more easily digested cooked. All of the raw salad vegetables, including broccoli and cauliflower flowerlets, (the tender parts of the vegetable), add much in the way of nutrition to the day's intake.

Hardier vegetables such as squash and potatoes (both sweet and white varieties) must be cooked to be completely palatable and digestible. Yoga does not favor extremes of food consumption; that is to say, Yoga maintains one should eat both raw foods and cooked ones. The composition of the food itself will dictate its method of preparation.

To some, the mention of meat summons up visions of steak, cutlets, chops, and other costly muscle meats. But better taste, greater nutrition, and more economical value can be had from the less popular organ meats. Heart, brains, kidneys, liver, sweetbreads, tongue, and tripe contain class A complete protein, rich in vitamins.

Dr. Benjamin S. Frank, New York physician and researcher in the field of degenerative diseases and the question of aging, uses nucleic acid therapy in his treatment of patients. Food rich in nucleic acid is brewer's yeast, fish (especially small sardines), herring roe, and organ meats.

Reclaiming Body Beauty Through Diet

For specific problems of the hair and skin, a dedicated person can begin a program of reclamation by planning a corrective diet, just as an organic farmer can reclaim poor soil by systematically putting nutrients back into the ground. Great changes can take place by the elimination of harmful foods, and the substitution of beauty foods.

There can be quick rewards with such a plan. The mapping of the campaign should be done with a knowledge of the body areas needing help, and of the foods which will supply the nutrients needed to rebuild those parts of the body.

For the millions of sufferers of oily, dry, or dandruffy hair, lank hair, hair without body, or splitting, slow growing hair, there is a definite aid and corrective measure to be found in the foods you eat. No food, whether good or bad, goes into your system without leaving evidence of its use somewhere on or in your body. If the food has been nourishing, then you profit by a zest for living, healthy hair, color in the face, strong shapely fingernails, and so forth.

If, on the other hand, the food was a rich pastry, a candy bar, a cup of coffee, a sugar-laden soft drink, or a plate of French fried potatoes, the opposite will be true. There may be a feeling of exhaustion, a loss of energy, a lack of lustre to the hair, paleness in the complexion, or a puffy, out-of-proportion body.

One of the first requirements for luxuriant hair growth is the elimination from the diet of excessive animal fats and carbohydrates. For anyone with hair problems, the removal of all greasy food and a reduction in starches is a vital step toward encouraging healthy hair growth.

Protein intake should be increased, preferably by eating more eggs, lean meats, poultry, fish, and cheese. B vitamins are essential to good hair growth, and brewer's yeast is an excellent source of the entire B complex family. Taking three tablespoons of yeast a day has helped many people achieve renewed hair growth, especially when the yeast supplement accompanied a completely revamped (and improved) diet.

Food deficiencies are quickly reflected in the skin. To reclaim or restore one's health, or even to bring about some minor improvement, Dr. Tom D. Spies, medical nutritionist, suggests an increase of protein to 120 grams or more a day. The Food and Nutrition Board of the National Research Council for Normal Health recommends 55-65 grams a day.)

This means that if you have been consuming 55 or 65 grams of protein a day, and problems of hair and skin have developed, it might be a good idea to step up your protein intake, in order to supply your body with the essentials for repair.

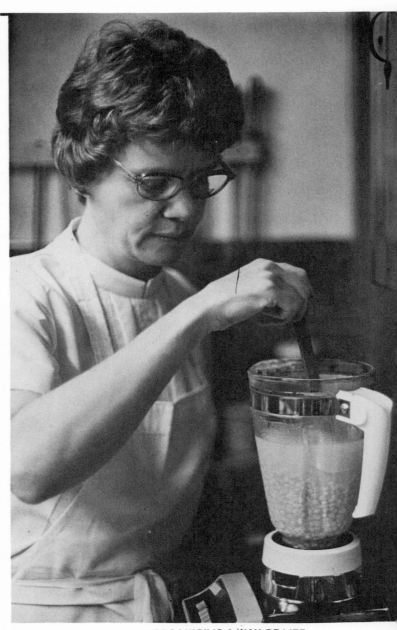

188

"ORGANIC" IS A WAY OF LIFE

In addition to the regular protein sources, a daily drink prepared in the blender is an easy and palatable way to add extra protein to the diet. This is an especially good method of protein supplementation for anyone who leads a busy life and cannot take time to prepare his own meals.

The blender is one piece of equipment that has become almost indispensable as a way of supplying beauty drinks with a minimum of effort. Such a drink can easily replace a complete meal on occasion. Many professional people have found that keeping a blender in the office, theater dressing room, or suitcase has helped them avoid the visible signs of age and exhaustion that come from too many lunch counter meals.

A favorite protein drink is made with two tablespoons of soya milk powder, two cups of water, a naturally fertilized egg yolk, one tablespoon of wheat germ, one table-spoon of sunflower meal, one tablespoon of unsulphured molasses, one apple, and two dates. This is all placed in the blender and liquidified and then drunk immediately as an excellent source of protein, and consequently, energy. The "side effects" are shining hair and good skin tone.

This drink can be varied in many ways, and the protein increased with the addition of a teaspoon of brewer's yeast. However, because of its strong taste, some find the addition of yeast objectionable. When this is the case, the yeast can always be rather successfully disguised in a glass of tomato juice.

Only fresh, nourishing foods can create the new cells that bring renewed life to the body facing an incredible barrage of irritations. If it is to manufacture healthy cells, the body must be treated as a garden, and nourished accordingly. If it isn't, the skin will dry, wrinkle, and age prematurely.

If the bloodstream that carries nourishment to every cell isn't able to carry away toxic wastes, then once again, one must turn to good nutrition. Special attention should be given to those foods which improve good blood circulation, thereby flushing accumulated wastes out of the body.

Daily intake of tomatoes, cucumbers, cabbage, parsley, watercress, cranberries, apples, or oranges will promote an inner cleansing activity that helps to prevent the muddying of the complexion that comes from a sluggish bloodstream.

In order to gain maximum benefit from beauty foods, draw up a list of food essentials and include them daily in the diet. Yoga teaches that life is a precious gift, to be nourished and cherished from beginning to end.

APPENDIX

RECIPES FOR BEAUTY AND HEALTH

SOUPS

Flemish Vegetable Soup

2 stalks celery
5 medium potatoes
1 cup tomato purée
2 small onions

1 tablespoon vegetable oil
1 clove garlic
pinch of thyme and chervil
1½ quarts water or stock

Dice the celery, potatoes, onions, and garlic and mix with tomato purée and water in a soup pot. Add the thyme, and salt to taste. Bring to a boil. Allow to cook over low heat until the vegetables are done. Strain and mash the vegetables, saving the liquid. Slowly add the liquid to make a rich, creamy mixture. Beat in the oil and serve.
Serves 4.

Pumpkin Soup

2 cups raw pumpkin,
   trimmed and chopped
2 cups water
1 teaspoon sea salt

2 tablespoons honey
4 cups soy milk
2 tablespoons nut oil

Simmer pumpkin, water, and salt in a large pot until soft. Strain, saving the liquid. Purée the pumpkin and beat in the cooking liquid. Return this mixture to pot. Add the honey and soy milk and simmer for five minutes. Remove from heat and beat in oil.
Serves 4.

Garbure Soup from the Pyrénées

2 tablespoons oil
3 carrots, diced
3 leeks, chopped
2 stalks celery, chopped
2 cups cabbage, chopped
1 teaspoon sea salt

3 cups water
3 cups consommé
3 small potatoes, chopped
1 cup cooked, dried white beans
1 cup green peas
   grated cheese

In a heavy pan, combine the first six ingredients. Cover and simmer over very low heat for thirty minutes. Add the water and consommé and bring to a boil. Add the potatoes, beans and peas and simmer until the vegetables are tender. Strain the vegetables, saving the liquid, and mash them through a sieve. Add the reserved liquid and mix well. Serve sprinkled with cheese.
Serves 4 to 6.

Potage St. Germain

1 leek or 1 onion
½ cup fresh green peas, cooked separately
2 cups marrowfat peas or navy beans, cooked
2 cups water or stock
6 spinach leaves

6 lettuce leaves
1 teaspoon sea salt
2 teaspoons honey
2 teaspoons oil
1 teaspoon chopped chervil

Coarsely mince the leek or onion and add to the chopped lettuce and spinach, the marrowfat peas, chervil, oil, salt, and one quarter cup of stock or water. Bring to a boil, lower the heat and simmer until the vegetables are tender before sieving them. Add the heated stock or water and the green peas after sieving. Serves 2 to 4.

Barley Soup

½ pound barley
2 ounces butter
1 leek or 1 onion
3 pints chicken stock

1 egg yolk

Cook the sliced white part of the leek, or the whole onion, in the butter until soft. Add chicken stock and barley and simmer until barley is done about ¾ hour. Sieve the barley and return to liquid. Beat the egg yolk with a little of the soup in a separate bowl and stir into the soup. Season to taste. Serves 4-6.

SALADS

Delta Salad

1 cup sprouts (mung, soya, radish, or other)
1 small green pepper (sweet)
1 small red pepper (sweet)
1 tablespoon lemon juice

2 teaspoons honey
2 tablespoons apple cider vinegar
1 small onion, sliced into rings

Steam sprouts and peppers together for five minutes. Drain. Prepare julienne strips of the peppers. Mix lemon juice, honey, and vinegar. Place sprouts, peppers, and onions in the sauce and toss until well-coated.

Radish and Mint Salad

2 cups sliced red radishes
1 small onion, chopped
2 small tomatoes, peeled, chopped
1 tablespoon fresh mint leaves. chopped

2 tablespoons lemon juice
¼ cup oil
1 teaspoon sea salt

Blend together oil, lemon juice, and sea salt. Combine tomatoes, onion, radishes, and mint leaves and pour oil dressing over them. Serve on shredded lettuce. Serves 4.

Carrot-Sesame Salad

2 cups grated carrots
½ cup green pepper, chopped
½ cup green onions, minced
½ cup celery, chopped
½ cup yogurt
toasted sesame seeds

Combine carrots, green pepper, onions and celery. Moisten with 2 teaspoons lemon juice, toss lightly with yogurt and sprinkle with toasted sesame seeds.

Garbanzo Salad

Mix 2 cups cooked garbanzos with ½ cup each of celery, green pepper, and onion. Shake together 6 tablespoons oil, 2 tablespoons lemon juice and ½ teaspoon sea salt with ½ teaspoon chopped thyme. Pour over vegetable mixture. Allow flavors to develop for an hour before serving.

Olla Podrida Salad

2 small apples
2 medium onions
6 tomatoes
2 boiled potatoes
1 tablespoon vinegar
2 tablespoons oil

2 hardboiled eggs
½ teaspoon sea salt

Rub a garlic clove around a salad bowl. Into the bowl, chop apples and onions fine. Chop 3 tomatoes, mixing the pulp with the apples and onions. Slice the potatoes thin and add to the salad with a mixture of the oil, vinegar, and salt. Let stand an hour and add the remaining tomatoes in slices, with the sliced eggs.

Beet and Carrot Salad

1 cup raw beets, grated
1 cup raw carrots, grated
1 cup radish sprouts
1 teaspoon crushed celery seeds

Mix together lightly. Use an oil and vinegar dressing.

Rice Salad Madras

2 cups cooked rice
4 tomatoes
2 green peppers
½ teaspoon sea salt
1 teaspoon minced oregano leaves
2 tablespoons oil

1 tablespoon apple cider vinegar
½ cup cooked shrimp

Peel and chop tomatoes. Cut peppers into short strips. In another bowl mix oil and vinegar. Add tomatoes, peppers, rice, and shrimp, stirring well after each addition. Allow to chill for one hour.
Serves 4.

LOOK YOUNGER - LOOK PRETTIER

Chicken Plov

1 broiler	*3 ounces butter*
2 ounces dried apricots	*1 tablespoon marigold petals*
2 ounces seedless raisins	*sea salt*
2 cups cooked brown rice	*water*

Soak the apricots and raisins in hot water for 2 hours. Pat dry on towelling and simmer in 1 ounce of butter until soft. Put rice into double boiler with 1 ounce of butter mixed with marigold petals. Stir well and cover. Allow to heat thoroughly. Separate chicken into four portions and rub seasoning all over the pieces. Sauté in remaining butter until browned on both sides. Arrange the chicken, rice, and fruit together for serving. Serves 4

Stuffed Grape Leaves

1 pound grape leaves	*1 tablespoon oil*
1 pound minced or ground lamb	*3 garlic cloves*
1 onion, chopped fine	*sea salt*
1 cup stock	*yogurt*

Mix the lamb, onion, rice, garlic, and salt together. Place the vine leaves into a shallow bowl of boiling water. Remove after a few minutes and pare away any of the hard part. Lay the leaves out flat and place one to two tablespoons of the meat mixture on each leaf. Carefully roll them up, tucking in the sides of the leaf to make a tight roll. Arrange the stuffed leaves close together in a casserole, sprinkle with salt and pour over them a mixture of the stock and the oil beaten together. Bake, covered, at 350 degrees for one hour. Serve with yogurt as an accompanying sauce.

Daube Glacé

2 pounds beef	*2 bay leaves*
2 onions	*2 sprigs thyme*
2 stalks celery	*2 tablespoons lemon juice*
2 cloves garlic	*2 tablespoons gelatin*
sea salt	*2 crushed egg shells*

Soak gelatin in one cup cold water. Gently simmer meat and seasoning in 3 quarts of water until liquid is reduced to 1 quart. Remove meat and chop into small pieces. Strain the liquid into a saucepan, add lemon juice and crushed egg shells. Boil together several minutes, until liquid is clarified. Strain and add to softened gelatin. Add the finely chopped meat to the gelatin liquid and pour into a loaf pan. Serves 10.

Broiled Kidneys

4 pairs lamb kidneys	*1 teaspoon sea salt*
1 tablespoon apple cider vinegar	*3 tablespoons oil*

Wash kidneys and cut in half lengthwise. Remove all fatty areas. Soak 15 minutes in cold water containing the salt and vinegar. Change water several times, adding salt and vinegar to each rinse. Drain, rinse under running water and dry thoroughly.

Dip kidneys in seasoned salad oil and place under broiler. Broil approximately 5 minutes on each side. Test doneness by cutting into thickest part of kidney. Serve with watercress, sliced tomatoes, and lemon slices. Serves 4.

Liver-Beef Loaf

1 pound beef liver, ground
1 onion, minced
½ cup celery, diced
¼ cup parsley, minced
3 tablespoons green pepper, minced
1 pound ground beef

2 tablespoons celery leaves, minced
1½ cups carrots, ground
½ cup wheat germ
2 eggs
½ cup stock or tomato juice
1 teaspoon sea salt

Mix all ingredients together and bake in a large, oiled loaf pan for one hour at 350 degrees. Serves 6 to 8.

Broiled Brains

2 pairs brains, precooked
2 tablespoons lemon juice

1 tablespoon oil
sea salt

Dip brains in mixture of lemon juice, oil and salt. Place on a broiling rack about 3 inches below the heat. Cook until delicately brown, 3 to 4 minutes on each side. Serve with chopped watercress dressed with lemon juice and oil.

Corfu Veal

1 cup cooked, minced veal
12 chopped almonds
1 egg

½ teaspoon sea salt
½ teaspoon oregano
1 cup tomato sauce

Mix meat, almonds, and seasonings and moisten with the well-beaten egg. Roll into balls the size of large walnuts and place in an oiled baking pan. Pour tomato sauce over them and bake for 20 minutes at 375 degrees. Serve over rice.

Marrow Balls

3 tablespoons marrow from young bones
4 tablespoons wheat germ
1 egg, beaten
½ teaspoon sea salt

½ teaspoon baking powder (from grapes)
⅛ teaspoon mace
1 tablespoon minced parsley

Beat marrow until creamy. Add remaining ingredients and blend. Chill until firm. Roll into small balls and drop in gently simmering soup. Cook for 10 minutes.

Mediterranean Fish Stew

1 lobster tail
½ pound fresh shrimp
½ pound cod
½ pound red snapper
½ pound bass
1 pound white fish filets
1 onion, minced
½ teaspoon saffron or marigold petals

⅓ cup olive oil
2 skinned and chopped tomatoes
2 garlic cloves, minced
1 sprig parsley
1 bay leaf
1 sprig thyme
1 sprig fennel

Cut the cleaned and boned fish into 2 inch pieces. Place the minced garlic, onions, and tomatoes into a pot along with the oil and herbs. Add the fish and cover with boiling water, no higher than the level of the fish. Bring to a boil, lower heat and simmer for 15 minutes. In serving, distribute a full variety of fish to each person. Serves 6-8.

Fish Kedgeree

1 cup cooked brown rice
1 cup flaked fish, cooked

1 tablespoon butter
1 egg

sea salt
chervil

Heat rice and fish in double boiler, stirring lightly. Add butter after mixture is heated, then the unbeaten egg, and seasoning. Stir until well-blended.

VEGETABLES AND EGGS

Lentil Roast

1 cup cooked lentils
1 cup chopped pecans
1 cup brown rice, cooked

1 cup soy milk
1 beaten egg
¼ cup oil

½ teaspoon crushed sage leaves
1 small chopped onion

Mix all ingredients together and bake at 350 degrees for 45 minutes.

Soybean Loaf

2 cups cooked soybeans
1 cup cooked brown rice
2 cups finely chopped walnuts
1 cup stock or soy milk

1 egg, beaten
1 tablespoon minced onion
1 tablespoon minced green pepper
1 teaspoon ground celery seeds

Mash beans and add to rice, nuts, milk, egg, onion, pepper, and crushed celery seeds. Mix together and pour into oiled loaf pan. Bake at 350 degrees for 1 hour. Serves 6.

Ratatouille - Mediterranean Vegetable Stew

6 medium onions
2 eggplants
3 zucchini

2 green peppers
3 tomatoes
bay leaf
parsley

tarragon
thyme
1 clove garlic

Slice all vegetables and brown onions, garlic, eggplants, zucchini, and green peppers in 4 tablespoons oil in heavy cast iron pan. Add remaining ingredients and cook 15 minutes longer. Place in a shallow baking dish and bake for one hour in a 325 degree oven. The volume decreases during baking. If there is too much liquid, remove the cover and allow to bake until liquid is lessened. Five minutes before serving, sprinkle grated cheese on top.

Piperade

1 large onion, chopped
2 sweet peppers, chopped
6 zucchini, sliced

1 tomato
6 eggs, beaten
parsley, chopped

chives, minced
3 tablespoons oil

Cook onion, pepper, zucchini, and tomato in oil in covered pan over a very low flame until done. Remove cover during the last five minutes to reduce moisture. Beat eggs and pour over mixture. Mix well to prevent scorching. Serve with parsley and chives.

Indian Kedgeree

2 cups brown rice
2 cups lentils

green ginger, sliced
bay leaf, cloves, sea salt

Soak lentils and rice for an hour and drain, saving liquid. Bring liquid to a boil, stir in all ingredients, and if needed, add water to cover. Lower heat and simmer in covered pot until tender.

Sweet Potato Loaf

1½ cups mashed sweet potatoes
3 ripe bananas, mashed
½ cup raisins
3 tablespoons raw sugar
¾ teaspoon sea salt

1 cup soy milk
⅓ teaspoon powdered nutmeg
⅓ teaspoon powdered cinnamon
3 eggs, beaten
½ cup grated nut meats

Combine sweet potatoes, bananas, milk, and sugar. Add sea salt, spices, and eggs. Mix thoroughly and pour into an oiled loaf pan. Sprinkle nutmeats over top and bake 1½ hours at 350 degrees.

Stuffed Turnips

6 medium sized turnips
2 onions, minced
¼ cup celery, chopped
¼ cup green pepper, minced
sea salt

1 cup ground beef
1 tablespoon oil
1 teaspoon sweet basil
¼ cup parsley, minced

Boil turnips until tender. Scoop out centers carefully. Sauté beef in oil, add celery, green pepper, and onions. Remove from heat and stir in parsley. Fill shells and sprinkle with wheat germ. Bake at 350 degrees for 20 minutes.

Corn Pudding

6 ears of fresh corn, grated
2 eggs, beaten separately

½ pint soy milk
sea salt

Beat whites of eggs. Add yolks to corn. Add milk and seasoning. Fold in egg whites very carefully and pour into an oiled loaf pan or casserole. Bake at 350 degrees for one hour.

Torino Eggplant

1 medium eggplant
3 tablespoons olive oil
2 garlic cloves

6 sprigs sweet basil
1 teaspoon crushed celery seeds
sea salt

Slice eggplant in half, lengthwise, and score. Insert small garlic pieces into each section of both halves. Rub the sweet basil into the olive oil with the crushed celery seeds and saturate the two halves with the herbed mixture. Salt to taste. Bake at 350 degrees until done.
Serves 2.

Corn Creole

2 cups fresh corn, grated
2 onions, minced
2 cloves garlic, minced
4 tablespoons butter

1 egg, beaten
2 cups soy milk
½ cup corn meal
salt to taste

Sauté onions and garlic in butter. Add corn, milk, and egg. Beat in corn meal and salt and cook in saucepan over low heat until thick, stirring constantly. Place in an oiled casserole and bake at 350 degrees for one hour.

Gazpacho

8 tomatoes, peeled, minced
2 onions, peeled, minced
3 cucumbers, peeled, minced
2 cloves garlic, peeled, minced
¼ cup olive oil

2 sweet green peppers, in strips
3 tablespoons apple cider vinegar
1½ cups tomato juice
½ cup minced parsley
2 teaspoons sea salt

Combine tomatoes, onions, cucumbers, peppers, and garlic in a deep bowl. Mix in olive oil, salt, vinegar, and tomato juice. Blend well. Cover tightly and refrigerate for three hours before using, to allow the flavors to blend.
Serves 4 to 6.

Curried Eggs and Sprouts

1 teaspoon butter
¼ cup finely chopped celery
⅛ cup chopped green pepper
½ teaspoon curry powder

3 beaten eggs
½ cup sprouts
  parsley

Melt butter in pan. Sauté celery and green peppers with curry powder until softened. Add beaten eggs and just before they are ready, add sprouts, mixing them about. Do not overcook the eggs. Garnish with parsley.

Cidracayote (Mexican Squash)

4 small summer squash, diced
1 teaspoon onion, minced
1 cup grated, fresh corn

1 tablespoon oil
½ teaspoon sea salt

Sauté squash and onions in oil. Cook for 10 minutes, stirring often. Add corn and cook until tender.

Dutch Red Cabbage

Cut a red cabbage into shreds and boil until tender. Drain as dry as possible and put into a pan with 2 tablespoons olive oil, 3 tablespoons apple cider vinegar and water, 1 minced onion, and ½ teaspoon sea salt. Allow to simmer until all the liquid evaporates.

Save the liquid in which the cabbage first boiled and use as a vitamin-rich drink.

DESSERTS

Strawberry Kissel

2 cups strawberries
½ cup honey

1 tablespoon potato flour
¾ pint water

Rub freshly washed and stemmed strawberries through a sieve. Bring water and honey to a boil in a saucepan. Blend a little of the liquid with the potato flour, pour into the saucepan and bring to a boil again. Pour the hot liquid over the puréed fruit and chill until serving time.

Kissel dessert can be made from a variety of fruits, such as raspberry, cherry, apple, plum, and cranberry. It can also be used as a sauce or dressing.

Georgian Fruit Rice Compote

½ cup stoned prunes
¼ cup raisins
¼ cup currants
½ cup chopped nutmeats

½ cup raw rice
2 tablespoons butter
2 tablespoons honey
water

Chop fruit and mix with nutmeats. Place in a saucepan with honey and enough water to cover. Simmer for 15 minutes. Boil rice until done. Pile pyramid style into bowl and pour compote over it.

Wheat Germ Brownies

4 eggs
2 cups brown sugar
2 tablespoons carob powder
1 teaspoon butter

2 teaspoons vanilla
2½ cups wheat germ
1 cup chopped nutmeats

Beat eggs, add sugar and beat together until light. Mix carob powder and butter. Add wheat germ, nutmeats, and vanilla. Bake in rectangular oiled pan at 375 degrees for 30 minutes. Cut into squares.

Carob-Lemon Cup Cakes

¼ cup oil
½ cup brown sugar
2 eggs, separated
⅓ cup soy milk

1 cup soya flour
1 teaspoon baking powder
2 tablespoons carob powder
2 teaspoon grated lemon peel

Cream oil and sugar together and add well-beaten egg yolks and lemon peel. Sift flour, baking powder, and carob powder together and add alternately with milk to first mixture. Fold in stiffly-beaten egg whites. Bake in muffin pans at 350 degrees until done.

Brown Rice Flour Muffins

1 cup brown rice flour
1½ teaspoons baking powder (from grapes)
¼ cup dark brown sugar
1 egg, beaten

¼ teaspoon sea salt
3 tablespoons oil
½ cup soy milk

Sift flour, baking powder, brown sugar, and salt together. Beat egg, milk, and oil together and fold into dry ingredients. Bake in an oiled muffin pan 15 minutes at 425 degrees.

Baked Prunes and Oranges in Honey

2 cups prunes
2 cups water
1 stick cinnamon
½ cup honey
1 orange

Soak prunes overnight in water. Next day bake at 350 degrees in tightly-covered casserole until tender. Add honey. Cut orange in thin slices and place on prunes. Cover and continue baking until orange slices are tender, about 45 minutes.

BREAKFAST CEREALS

Muesli - Breakfast Cereal

2 cups finely chopped oats
½ cup chopped nutmeats, soaked for
several hours beforehand
2 grated apples, skins included

2 tablespoons raisins
juice of ½ orange
1 tablespoon honey
1 cup soy milk

Mix together and soak overnight. Use as a breakfast cereal.

Ready-Mix Breakfast Cereal

½ cup sunflower seed meal
½ cup pumpkin seed meal
1 cup wheat germ

½ cup finely chopped nutmeats
½ cup soy flakes
½ cup chopped apricots

Mix together well and keep in closed container in refrigerator until ready to use. Use with soy or seed milk.

MILKS

Coconut Milk

2 cups freshly grated coconut
2 cups warm water

1 tablespoon honey
pinch of sea salt

Liquify for two minutes in blender and strain.

Sesame Seed Milk

¼ cup sesame seed
1½ cups water
1 tablespoon honey

Liquify for two minutes in blender and strain to remove hulls.

Soy Date Milk

½ cup soy powder
1 cup water
3 dates

Liquify the soy powder and water for two minutes in blender. Add the dates and liquify for another two minutes, until well blended.

Grateful acknowledgement is hereby made for photography by A. Devany, Inc., N.Y.N.Y.; H. Armstrong Roberts, Philadelphia, Pa.; Harold Lambert Studios, Philadelphia, Pa.; David Gooley & Associates, Paramount, Cal.; and Rodale Press Photo Lab. Illustrations by Jean Bargeron and Joseph Charnoski, Retouching by William Rathgeber.
Jacket design, Susan Heagy.

LOOK YOUNGER - LOOK PRETTIER